HOW TO GET RID OF BACK PAIN IN 2024

BY:

MARK BARNETT

Introduction

Welcome to "HOW TO GET RID OF BACK PAIN IN 2024," your comprehensive guide to understanding and managing back pain effectively. Whether you've recently experienced back discomfort or have been coping with chronic pain, this book aims to equip you with practical strategies and insights to regain control over your back health.

Back pain can be disruptive, impacting your daily activities, work, and overall well-being. However, it doesn't have to define your life. With the right knowledge, personalized approaches, and a proactive mindset, it's possible to alleviate pain, regain function, and enhance your quality of life.

In the following chapters, we'll explore various aspects of back pain management, focusing on creating a personalized plan tailored to your unique needs. From understanding the causes of back pain to practical exercises, lifestyle adjustments, and seeking professional guidance, this book will provide you with valuable tools and resources to navigate your journey towards a healthier back.

We encourage you to approach this book as your companion in your pursuit of a pain-free life. By delving into these pages and implementing the suggested strategies, you'll discover ways to effectively manage your back pain, regain strength, and restore your vitality.

Let's embark on this journey together, empowering you to take charge of your back health and embrace a life free from the limitations imposed by back pain.

Title: "How To Get Rid Of Back Pain In 2024"

Understanding Back Pain Causes

Importance of Proper Posture

Core Strengthening Exercises

Stretching and Flexibility Routines

Ergonomic Adjustments in Daily Life

Importance of Weight Management

Pain Relief through Hot and Cold Therapy

Incorporating Low-Impact Aerobic Exercises

Mind-Body Techniques for Relaxation

Guidance on Proper Lifting Techniques

Role of Good Sleep in Back Health

Benefits of Massage Therapy

Dietary Changes for Back Pain Relief

Seeking Professional Medical Advice

Exploring Over-the-Counter Medications

Understanding the Role of Stress in Back Pain

Trying Acupuncture or Acupressure

Chiropractic Care for Back Pain

Benefits of Physical Therapy

Using Lumbar Support Pillows or Cushions

Yoga and its Impact on Back Health

Pilates Exercises for Core Strength

Hydrotherapy and Water-Based Exercises

Cognitive Behavioral Therapy for Pain Management

Supportive Shoe Choices and Footwear

Role of Inflammation in Back Pain

Workplace Ergonomics and Back Health

Mindfulness and Meditation Practices

Tai Chi for Balance and Flexibility

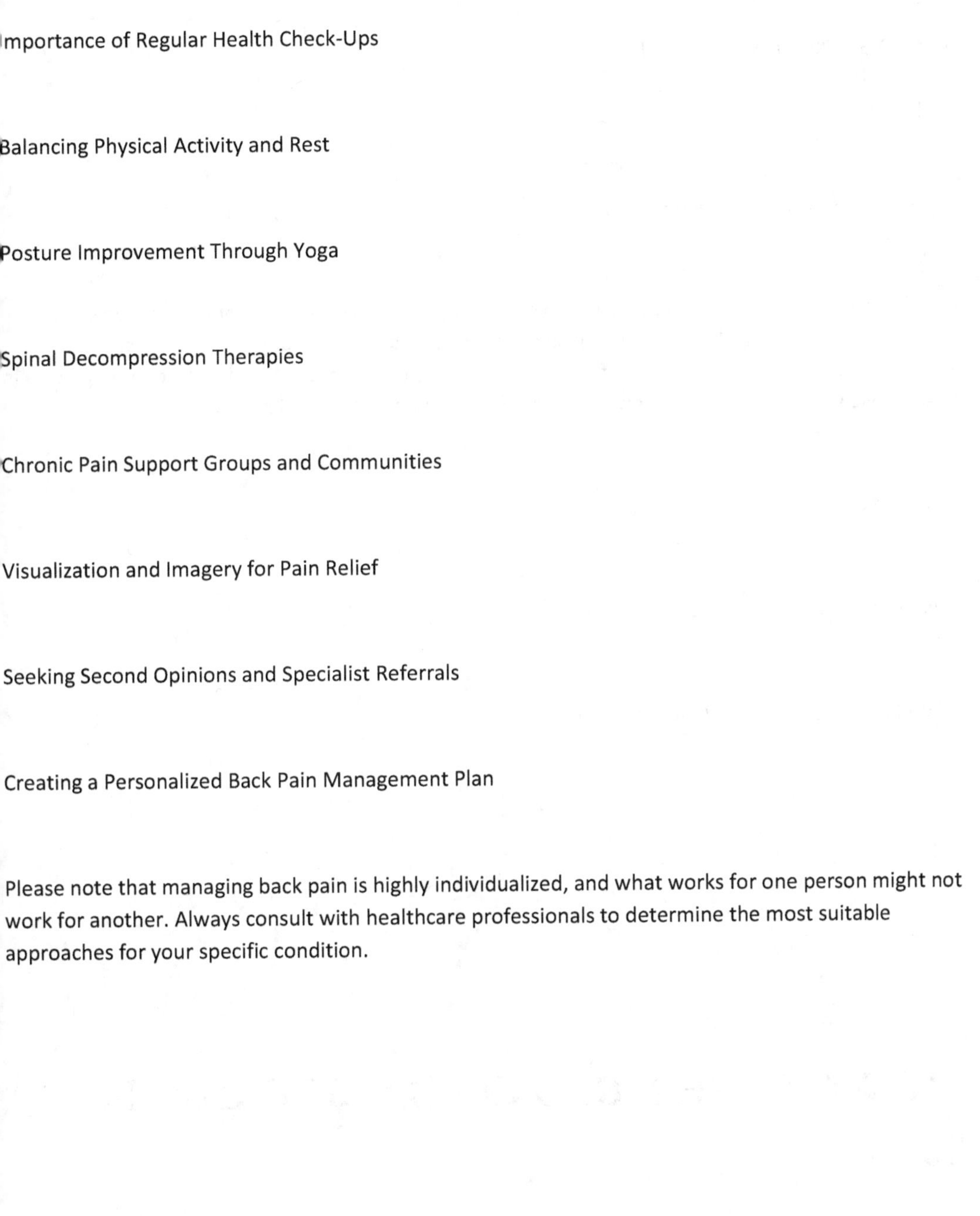

Importance of Regular Health Check-Ups

Balancing Physical Activity and Rest

Posture Improvement Through Yoga

Spinal Decompression Therapies

Chronic Pain Support Groups and Communities

Visualization and Imagery for Pain Relief

Seeking Second Opinions and Specialist Referrals

Creating a Personalized Back Pain Management Plan

Please note that managing back pain is highly individualized, and what works for one person might not work for another. Always consult with healthcare professionals to determine the most suitable approaches for your specific condition.

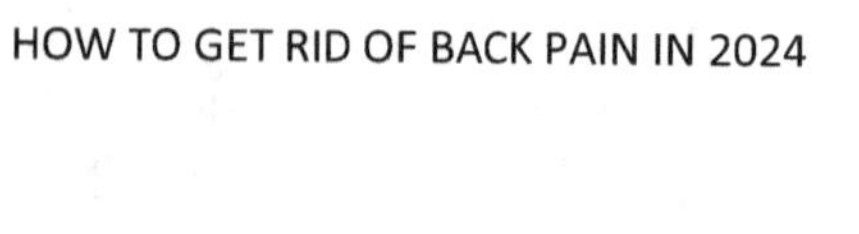

HOW TO GET RID OF BACK PAIN IN 2024

CHAPTER 1

Understanding the causes of back pain can help in finding ways to manage and prevent it. While back pain can be caused by various factors, here's an explanation of some common causes:

Muscle or Ligament Strain: Back pain often results from overstretching or tearing of muscles or ligaments due to sudden movements, lifting heavy objects, or poor posture.

Disc Problems: Issues with the spinal discs, like herniation or bulging discs, can press on nerves, leading to back pain. This may occur due to aging or injuries.

Spinal Stenosis: Narrowing of the spinal canal due to wear and tear over time can exert pressure on the spinal cord and nerves, causing pain.

Arthritis: Osteoarthritis or other forms of arthritis can affect the spine, leading to pain, stiffness, and decreased mobility.

Scoliosis: An abnormal curvature of the spine can cause discomfort or pain due to uneven pressure on the spinal structures.

Osteoporosis: Weakening of bones, especially in older adults, can result in fractures in the spine, causing pain and reduced mobility.

Traumatic Injuries: Accidents, falls, or injuries can lead to fractures, sprains, or strains, causing acute or chronic back pain.

Underlying Health Conditions: Back pain might be a symptom of other health issues like kidney stones, infections, or tumors affecting the spine.

Poor Posture and Lifestyle: Prolonged sitting, incorrect posture while standing or lifting heavy objects, obesity, and lack of exercise can strain the back muscles and lead to pain.

To manage or prevent back pain, maintaining a healthy lifestyle, practicing good posture, regular exercise to strengthen core muscles, proper lifting techniques, and seeking medical advice when needed are crucial steps. Remember, every individual's situation is unique, so consulting healthcare professionals for personalized advice is essential for effective back pain management.

CHAPTER 2

Understanding Proper Posture:

What is Proper Posture?

Proper posture involves maintaining the body in a position where the least strain is placed on muscles, ligaments, and joints while standing, sitting, or lying down.

Importance of Good Posture:

Spinal Alignment: Correct posture keeps the spine properly aligned, reducing stress on the vertebrae and minimizing the risk of back pain, stiffness, and discomfort.

Muscle Balance: It helps distribute body weight evenly, preventing excessive strain on specific muscles and avoiding muscle imbalances that could lead to pain.

Improved Breathing: Good posture allows the lungs to expand fully, promoting better breathing and oxygen intake, which is essential for overall health.

Enhanced Digestion: Proper posture aids in optimal digestion by allowing organs in the abdomen to function without unnecessary compression, preventing digestive issues.

Prevention of Joint Degeneration: Maintaining correct alignment decreases wear and tear on joints, potentially reducing the risk of joint problems as one ages.

Tips for Maintaining Good Posture:

Standing: Keep your head up, shoulders back, and spine straight. Distribute body weight evenly on both feet, and avoid locking knees.

Sitting: Sit upright with your back against the chair, feet flat on the floor, and knees at or below hip level. Use a chair with proper lumbar support.

Sleeping: Choose a mattress and pillow that support the natural curvature of your spine and sleep in positions that align the spine, like on your side with knees slightly bent.

Lifting: Bend your knees and keep your back straight while lifting objects. Hold items close to your body and avoid twisting when lifting.

Screen Time: Position screens at eye level to avoid neck strain. Take regular breaks to stretch and move if sitting for extended periods.

Incorporating Good Posture Into Daily Life:

Making small adjustments to daily habits can help maintain good posture:

Stay mindful of your posture throughout the day.

Perform exercises to strengthen core muscles, supporting the spine.

Use ergonomic furniture and equipment that promotes good posture.

Consider posture-correcting devices or reminders to maintain alignment.

Conclusion:

Practicing proper posture is fundamental in preventing back pain, reducing strain on muscles and joints, and supporting overall health. By being mindful of posture and making necessary adjustments, individuals can significantly improve their well-being and minimize the risk of discomfort and pain associated with poor posture.

CHAPTER 3

Understanding Core Strength:

What is the Core?

The core comprises muscles in the abdomen, lower back, pelvis, and hips that work together to provide stability, support, and balance to the body.

Importance of Core Strength:

Spinal Support: A strong core stabilizes the spine, reducing the risk of back pain by supporting proper posture and alignment.

mproved Balance and Stability: Core strength enhances balance, stability, and coordination, reducing the likelihood of falls or injuries.

Enhanced Athletic Performance: Athletes benefit from a strong core as it aids in generating power, improving performance in various sports or physical activities.

Reduced Risk of Injury: Strong core muscles provide better support to the entire body during movements, lowering the risk of strains or overuse injuries.

Better Functional Movement: A strong core enables easier and more efficient movement in daily activities, such as bending, lifting, and reaching.

Simple Core Strengthening Exercises:

Plank:

Start on the floor with elbows directly beneath the shoulders.

Raise your body, keeping it in a straight line from head to heels.

Hold the position for 20-30 seconds initially and gradually increase as strength improves.

Bridge:

Lie on your back with knees bent and feet flat on the floor.

Lift your hips off the ground, creating a straight line from shoulders to knees.

Hold for a few seconds before lowering down.

Leg Raises:

Lie on your back with legs straight.

Slowly lift both legs together to a 45-degree angle, then lower them back down without touching the floor.

Russian Twists:

Sit on the floor, knees bent, and feet flat.

Lean back slightly, engage your core, and twist your torso from side to side, touching the floor near your hips.

Bird Dog:

Get on all fours, keeping your back straight.

Extend one arm forward and the opposite leg backward while keeping the hips stable.

Return to the starting position and switch sides.

Incorporating Core Exercises:

Aim for regular workouts, starting with a few repetitions and gradually increasing as strength improves.

Perform core exercises at least 2-3 times a week.

Combine with cardiovascular exercises and a balanced diet for overall fitness.

Consult a fitness professional or physiotherapist for guidance on suitable exercises.

Conclusion:

Core strengthening exercises are vital for maintaining a strong and stable core, supporting spine health, preventing injuries, and improving overall fitness and functionality in daily life. Incorporating these simple exercises into a regular routine can significantly benefit individuals in achieving better core strength and overall well-being.

CHAPTER 4

Understanding Stretching and Flexibility:

What is Stretching?

Stretching involves gently lengthening muscles to improve flexibility, range of motion, and muscle elasticity.

Importance of Stretching:

Enhanced Flexibility: Regular stretching helps increase flexibility, allowing joints to move through their full range of motion and reducing muscle tension.

Injury Prevention: Improved flexibility reduces the risk of strains, sprains, and muscle injuries by preparing muscles and joints for movement.

Improved Posture: Stretching exercises can help correct muscle imbalances and promote better posture by releasing tension in tight muscles.

Reduced Muscle Soreness: Stretching after exercise can alleviate muscle soreness and stiffness by promoting blood flow and aiding in muscle recovery.

Stress Relief: Stretching relaxes muscles and can provide stress relief, promoting relaxation and a sense of well-being.

Simple Stretching and Flexibility Exercises:

Hamstring Stretch:

Sit on the floor with one leg extended and the other bent.

Lean forward, reaching toward your toes while keeping your back straight.

Calf Stretch:

Stand facing a wall, with one foot forward and the other back.

Lean forward, keeping the back leg straight and the heel on the ground.

Quadriceps Stretch:

Stand upright and bring one foot up toward your buttocks, holding the ankle behind you.

Gently pull the foot toward the buttocks while keeping the knees close together.

Shoulder Stretch:

Stand or sit tall, and bring one arm across your body.

Use the opposite hand to gently pull the arm closer to your chest, feeling a stretch in the shoulder.

Trunk Rotation:

Sit on the floor with legs extended.

Twist your torso to one side, placing the opposite arm on the outside of the bent knee for a gentle stretch.

Incorporating Stretching into Daily Routine:

Perform stretching exercises at least 2-3 times a week, aiming for consistency.

Warm up your body with light activity before stretching to increase effectiveness.

Hold each stretch for 15-30 seconds, avoiding bouncing or jerking movements.

Breathe deeply and relax into each stretch, avoiding pain or discomfort.

Conclusion:

Regular stretching and flexibility exercises are essential for improving flexibility, reducing the risk of injury, promoting relaxation, and enhancing overall well-being. By incorporating these simple stretching routines into a regular schedule, individuals can enjoy increased flexibility, improved mobility, and a more relaxed and comfortable body.

CHAPTER 5

Understanding Ergonomics:

What is Ergonomics?

Ergonomics focuses on designing and arranging the environment to fit the needs of the individual, aiming to reduce discomfort, fatigue, and stress on the body.

Importance of Ergonomic Adjustments:

Improved Posture: Ergonomic adjustments promote proper body alignment, reducing strain on muscles and joints, which helps prevent back, neck, and shoulder pain.

Reduced Fatigue: Properly designed workspaces or environments that support ergonomic principles can reduce physical and mental fatigue, enhancing productivity and comfort.

Prevention of Musculoskeletal Issues: Ergonomic adjustments can mitigate the risk of repetitive strain injuries or musculoskeletal disorders caused by prolonged poor posture or uncomfortable positions.

Enhanced Comfort and Well-Being: Implementing ergonomic solutions in daily life enhances comfort, supporting better concentration, focus, and overall well-being.

Simple Ergonomic Adjustments:

Workspace Ergonomics:

Ensure your chair supports the lower back and allows feet to rest flat on the floor or on a footrest.

Position the computer monitor at eye level to reduce strain on the neck and eyes.

Keep frequently used items within easy reach to avoid excessive stretching or reaching.

Proper Lifting Techniques:

Bend at the knees, not the waist, when lifting heavy objects to reduce strain on the back.

Hold objects close to your body and avoid twisting while lifting.

Adjusting Sleeping Posture:

Use a pillow that supports the natural curve of the neck while sleeping to maintain spinal alignment.

Experiment with different mattresses to find one that offers proper support.

Ergonomic Furniture:

Choose chairs, desks, and other furniture that support good posture and provide proper body support.

Breaks and Movement:

Take frequent breaks from prolonged sitting or repetitive tasks to stretch and move around.

Incorporate stretching exercises or short walks into the daily routine to reduce stiffness.

Incorporating Ergonomic Principles:

Make small adjustments to workspaces, chairs, or equipment to promote better posture and comfort.

Be mindful of body positioning and take regular breaks to avoid prolonged periods in one position.

Consult ergonomic specialists or occupational therapists for personalized advice on ergonomic adjustments.

Conclusion:

Implementing ergonomic adjustments in daily life, whether at work or home, can significantly improve posture, reduce discomfort, and enhance overall well-being. By making simple changes to support proper body alignment and reduce strain, individuals can enjoy increased comfort and productivity while minimizing the risk of musculoskeletal issues.

CHAPTER 6

Understanding Weight Management:

What is Weight Management?

Weight management involves adopting healthy habits to achieve and maintain a healthy weight range through a balanced diet, regular exercise, and lifestyle changes.

Importance of Weight Management:

Overall Health Improvement: Maintaining a healthy weight reduces the risk of various health conditions, including heart disease, diabetes, high blood pressure, and certain cancers.

Joint Health: Excess weight places additional stress on joints, leading to increased wear and tear, discomfort, and a higher risk of joint problems like osteoarthritis.

Reduced Risk of Chronic Conditions: Maintaining a healthy weight can lower the risk of chronic conditions, improving overall quality of life and reducing the need for medication.

Improved Energy Levels: Achieving and maintaining a healthy weight can enhance energy levels and reduce feelings of fatigue and lethargy.

Enhanced Self-Esteem: Managing weight contributes to a positive body image, boosting self-confidence

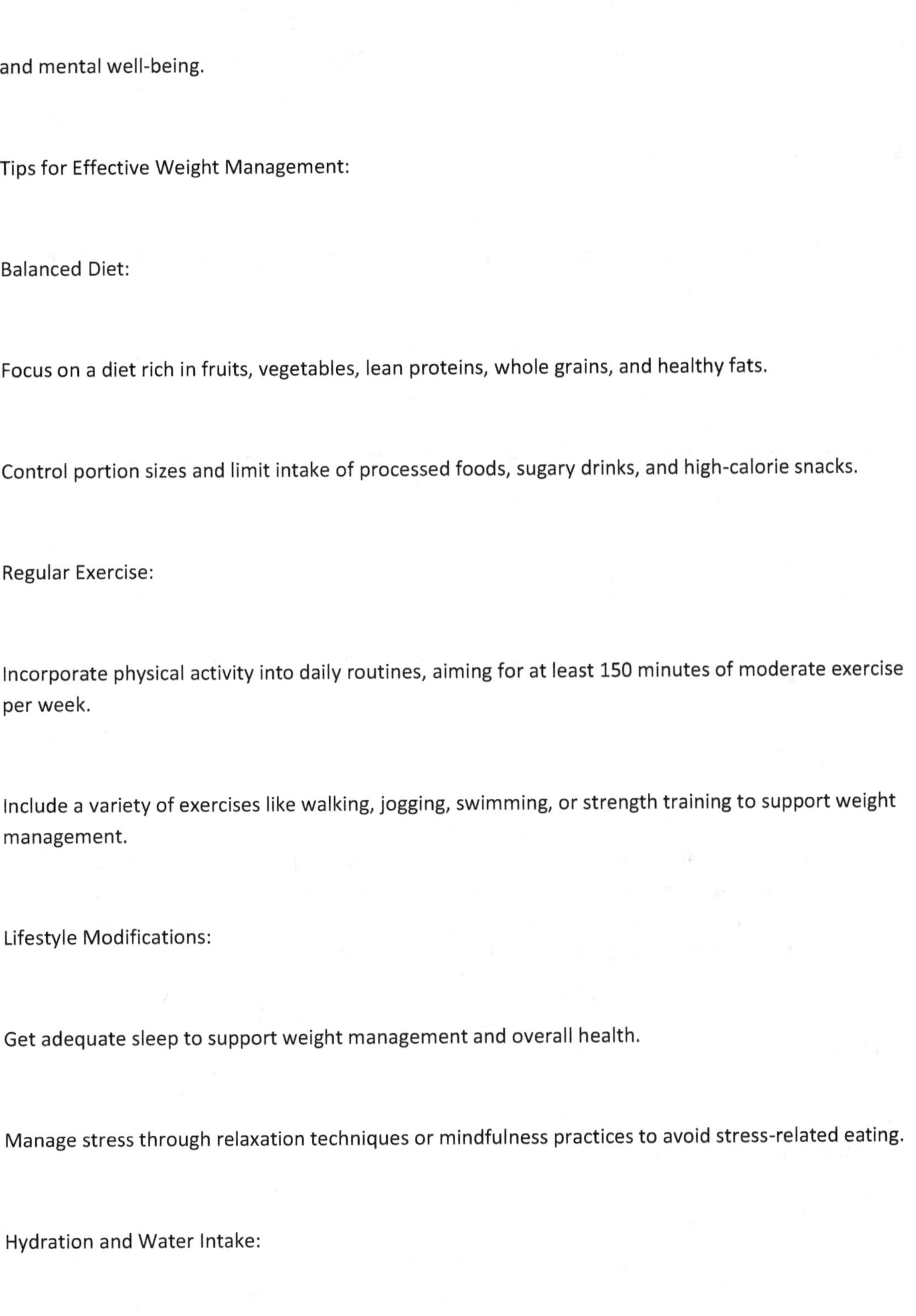

and mental well-being.

Tips for Effective Weight Management:

Balanced Diet:

Focus on a diet rich in fruits, vegetables, lean proteins, whole grains, and healthy fats.

Control portion sizes and limit intake of processed foods, sugary drinks, and high-calorie snacks.

Regular Exercise:

Incorporate physical activity into daily routines, aiming for at least 150 minutes of moderate exercise per week.

Include a variety of exercises like walking, jogging, swimming, or strength training to support weight management.

Lifestyle Modifications:

Get adequate sleep to support weight management and overall health.

Manage stress through relaxation techniques or mindfulness practices to avoid stress-related eating.

Hydration and Water Intake:

Drink plenty of water throughout the day to stay hydrated and support metabolic processes.

Seeking Professional Guidance:

Consult with healthcare professionals or registered dietitians for personalized advice and support.

Incorporating Healthy Habits:

Make gradual changes to eating habits and exercise routines for sustainable weight management.

Set realistic goals and track progress to stay motivated on the weight management journey.

Focus on overall health and well-being rather than just the number on the scale.

Conclusion:

Effective weight management is crucial for overall health, reducing the risk of chronic diseases, improving energy levels, and enhancing self-esteem. By adopting healthy eating habits, incorporating regular physical activity, and making lifestyle changes, individuals can achieve and maintain a healthy weight, leading to a better quality of life and improved overall well-being.

CHAPTER 7

Understanding Hot and Cold Therapy:

What is Hot and Cold Therapy?

Hot and cold therapy involves using temperature-based treatments to alleviate pain, reduce inflammation, and promote healing in injured or sore areas of the body.

Importance of Hot and Cold Therapy:

Pain Relief: Alternating between hot and cold treatments can alleviate different types of pain, including muscle aches, strains, sprains, and joint discomfort.

Reduction of Inflammation: Cold therapy helps constrict blood vessels, reducing inflammation and swelling in injured areas, while heat improves blood flow, aiding in healing.

Muscle Relaxation: Heat therapy relaxes muscles, easing stiffness and tension, while cold therapy numbs the area, providing relief from acute pain.

Injury Recovery: Hot and cold treatments can accelerate the recovery process by improving blood circulation and promoting tissue healing.

Types of Hot and Cold Therapy:

Cold Therapy:

Applying ice packs, cold packs, or frozen gel packs to the affected area for 15-20 minutes at a time, multiple times a day, within the first 48 hours of an injury.

Heat Therapy:

Using heating pads, warm towels, or warm baths to apply gentle heat to the affected area for 15-20 minutes, promoting relaxation and reducing muscle tension.

When to Use Hot or Cold Therapy:

Cold Therapy is beneficial for acute injuries, such as sprains, strains, or bruises, as it reduces swelling and numbs pain.

Heat Therapy is more suitable for chronic conditions or to alleviate stiffness, as it promotes blood flow and relaxes muscles.

Precautions and Tips:

Always use a barrier (like a cloth or towel) between the skin and hot or cold packs to avoid skin damage.

Limit application time to prevent skin irritation or burns.

Avoid using heat on areas with swelling, and refrain from using cold therapy for more than 20 minutes at a time to prevent frostbite.

Conclusion:

Hot and cold therapy are effective and easy-to-use methods for relieving pain, reducing inflammation, and aiding in the healing process for various injuries and discomforts. By understanding when and how to apply these therapies, individuals can effectively manage pain and support the recovery of sore or injured areas, contributing to overall comfort and well-being.

CHAPTER 8

Understanding Low-Impact Aerobic Exercises:

What are Low-Impact Aerobic Exercises?

Low-impact aerobic exercises are activities that raise the heart rate and increase breathing without subjecting the body to excessive stress or strain.

Importance of Low-Impact Aerobic Exercises:

Cardiovascular Health: Low-impact aerobics improve heart health by strengthening the heart and enhancing circulation, reducing the risk of heart disease and stroke.

Weight Management: These exercises help burn calories, supporting weight loss or weight maintenance goals, without excessive impact on joints.

Joint Health: They are gentle on joints, making them suitable for individuals with joint pain, arthritis, or those recovering from injuries.

Improved Endurance and Stamina: Regular participation in low-impact aerobics can enhance endurance, stamina, and overall energy levels.

Mental Well-Being: These exercises release endorphins, boosting mood, reducing stress, and promoting a sense of well-being.

Types of Low-Impact Aerobic Exercises:

Walking: Brisk walking is an excellent low-impact exercise that can be easily incorporated into daily routines.

Swimming: Swimming or water aerobics provide a full-body workout while minimizing stress on joints.

Cycling: Stationary or outdoor cycling is a low-impact exercise that strengthens leg muscles and improves cardiovascular health.

Elliptical Training: Using an elliptical machine at the gym offers a low-impact cardio workout for the whole body.

Dancing: Dance-based workouts or low-impact dance classes can be enjoyable while providing aerobic benefits.

Incorporating Low-Impact Aerobics into Daily Routine:

Start slowly and gradually increase the duration and intensity of workouts.

Aim for at least 150 minutes of moderate-intensity aerobic exercise per week, following guidelines from health professionals.

Incorporate variety into workouts to prevent boredom and engage different muscle groups.

Safety Precautions:

Listen to your body and stop exercising if you experience pain or discomfort.

Wear appropriate footwear and comfortable clothing while exercising.

Consult a healthcare provider before starting any exercise program, especially if you have health concerns or medical conditions.

Conclusion:

Low-impact aerobic exercises offer numerous health benefits, including improved cardiovascular health, weight management, joint support, increased stamina, and mental well-being. By incorporating these gentle yet effective exercises into regular routines, individuals can enjoy the advantages of aerobic workouts while minimizing stress on the body, fostering overall health and fitness.

CHAPTER 9

Understanding Mind-Body Techniques for Relaxation:

What are Mind-Body Techniques?

Mind-body techniques involve practices that link mental focus, breathing, and physical movements to promote relaxation, reduce stress, and improve overall well-being.

Importance of Mind-Body Techniques:

Stress Reduction: Mind-body techniques aid in reducing stress levels by calming the mind and relaxing the body's physiological responses to stressors.

Improved Mental Health: These techniques can alleviate symptoms of anxiety, depression, and mood disorders, promoting mental clarity and emotional balance.

Enhanced Physical Health: Relaxation techniques may help lower blood pressure, improve sleep quality, and boost the immune system, contributing to better physical health.

Pain Management: They can complement pain management strategies by reducing muscle tension and promoting relaxation in areas of discomfort.

Overall Well-Being: Regular practice of mind-body techniques fosters a sense of inner peace, mindfulness, and a greater connection between the mind and body.

Types of Mind-Body Techniques:

Deep Breathing Exercises: Techniques like diaphragmatic breathing or abdominal breathing promote relaxation by slowing down the breath and activating the body's relaxation response.

Meditation: Meditation involves focusing the mind, often using breath awareness or guided imagery, to promote relaxation and mental clarity.

Progressive Muscle Relaxation (PMR): PMR involves tensing and then relaxing different muscle groups systematically, reducing muscle tension and inducing relaxation.

Yoga: Yoga combines physical postures, breathing exercises, and meditation to enhance flexibility, balance, and relaxation.

Tai Chi: Tai Chi involves slow, flowing movements, promoting relaxation, balance, and mental focus.

Incorporating Mind-Body Techniques into Daily Routine:

Set aside a specific time each day for relaxation practice.

Start with short sessions and gradually increase duration as comfort and skill improve.

Experiment with different techniques to find the ones that resonate best with personal preferences.

Safety Precautions:

Practice mind-body techniques in a quiet, safe environment.

If following instructional videos or guides, ensure they come from reputable sources.

If experiencing severe stress or mental health concerns, seek guidance from a mental health professional.

Conclusion:

Mind-body techniques offer powerful tools for relaxation, stress reduction, and overall well-being. By incorporating these practices into daily routines, individuals can experience the benefits of relaxation, such as reduced stress levels, improved mental and physical health, and a greater sense of calm and balance in their lives.

CHAPTER 10

Understanding Proper Lifting Techniques:

Why are Proper Lifting Techniques Important?

Proper lifting techniques are crucial to prevent injuries and strain on the body while moving or lifting objects.

Importance of Proper Lifting Techniques:

Injury Prevention: Using correct lifting methods reduces the risk of back injuries, strains, sprains, and muscle pulls.

Spinal Health: Proper techniques protect the spine by minimizing stress on the back muscles, discs, and ligaments.

Efficient Movement: Applying correct lifting techniques makes lifting easier and more efficient, allowing for better use of muscle strength.

Reduced Muscle Fatigue: Employing the right methods prevents unnecessary strain on muscles, reducing fatigue and discomfort.

Guidelines for Proper Lifting:

Plan and Assess:

Before lifting, assess the object's weight, size, and position. Plan your approach and the path you will take.

Use Proper Form:

Bend at the knees, not the waist, keeping your back straight and chest forward.

Keep the object close to your body as you lift.

Lift with Your Legs:

Use the power of your leg muscles by squatting to the object's level and lifting with your legs while keeping your back straight.

Avoid Twisting:

Turn your entire body instead of twisting at the waist when carrying the object.

Steady Movement:

Lift and lower the object slowly and smoothly, avoiding sudden or jerky movements.

Additional Tips:

Assistance: For heavy or bulky objects, seek help or use lifting aids like dollies or carts.

Break Down Loads: If possible, divide heavy loads into smaller, manageable parts to lift.

Footwear: Wear proper footwear with good traction to prevent slipping or losing balance.

Safety Precautions:

Always ask for help with heavy or awkward objects, especially if unsure about lifting them safely.

Avoid lifting immediately after prolonged periods of inactivity or if feeling fatigued.

Conclusion:

Proper lifting techniques are essential for preventing injuries, protecting spinal health, and ensuring efficient movement. By following these simple guidelines and prioritizing safety when lifting objects, individuals can significantly reduce the risk of strain or injury, promoting a safer and healthier lifestyle.

CHAPTER 11

Understanding the Role of Good Sleep in Back Health:

Why is Good Sleep Important for Back Health?

Quality sleep plays a vital role in supporting back health by allowing the body to repair, rejuvenate, and maintain overall well-being.

Importance of Good Sleep for Back Health:

Muscle Relaxation: During sleep, muscles relax, allowing the back muscles to recover from daily stress and tension.

Tissue Repair: Adequate sleep supports tissue repair, including the healing of damaged back tissues and muscles.

Spinal Alignment: Sleep allows the spine to rest in a neutral position, reducing strain on the back and supporting proper spinal alignment.

Pain Management: Quality sleep can alleviate back pain by reducing inflammation and promoting the release of natural pain-relieving substances.

Mental Health: Poor sleep affects mood and mental health, potentially exacerbating back pain due to increased stress and tension.

Tips for Improving Sleep for Better Back Health:

Establish a Sleep Routine:

Aim for a consistent sleep schedule by going to bed and waking up at the same time every day, even on weekends.

Create a Relaxing Environment:

Ensure the sleep environment is comfortable, quiet, and dark, promoting relaxation and uninterrupted sleep.

Supportive Sleep Surface:

Choose a mattress and pillows that provide proper support for the back, promoting spinal alignment and reducing pressure points.

Limit Screen Time Before Bed:

Avoid electronic devices like phones and computers before bedtime, as the blue light emitted can disrupt sleep patterns.

Regular Physical Activity:

Engage in regular exercise to promote better sleep quality and reduce stress, contributing to improved back health.

Healthy Sleep Habits:

Avoid heavy meals, caffeine, and alcohol close to bedtime.

Practice relaxation techniques such as deep breathing or meditation to unwind before sleep.

If experiencing sleep problems or persistent back pain, consult with a healthcare professional.

Conclusion:

Quality sleep is essential for maintaining good back health. By prioritizing good sleep habits, establishing a consistent sleep routine, and creating a comfortable sleep environment, individuals can support their back health, reduce back pain, and improve overall well-being.

CHAPTER 12

Understanding the Benefits of Massage Therapy:

What is Massage Therapy?

Massage therapy involves the manipulation of soft tissues in the body to alleviate tension, promote relaxation, and improve overall well-being.

Importance of Massage Therapy:

Stress Reduction: Massage therapy helps reduce stress by relaxing muscles and promoting the release of feel-good hormones like serotonin and dopamine.

Pain Relief: It can alleviate muscle tension, reduce discomfort, and ease chronic pain conditions such as back pain, headaches, and arthritis.

Improved Circulation: Massage increases blood flow, enhancing oxygen and nutrient delivery to tissues and aiding in the removal of metabolic waste.

Enhanced Flexibility and Range of Motion: Regular massages can improve flexibility, joint mobility, and reduce stiffness, promoting better physical performance.

Mental Well-being: Massage therapy can reduce anxiety, depression, and improve sleep quality, contributing to overall mental health.

Types of Massage Therapy and Their Benefits:

Swedish Massage:

Benefits: Relaxation, stress reduction, improved circulation.

Deep Tissue Massage:

Benefits: Alleviates chronic muscle tension, reduces pain, improves flexibility.

Sports Massage:

Benefits: Enhances athletic performance, aids in injury prevention and recovery.

Trigger Point Therapy:

Benefits: Targets specific points of muscle tension, reducing pain and improving mobility.

Incorporating Massage Therapy into Wellness Routine:

Schedule regular massages based on personal needs and preferences.

Communicate openly with the massage therapist about preferences, pain areas, and desired pressure.

Safety Precautions:

Inform the massage therapist about any health conditions, injuries, or discomfort before the session.

Ensure the massage therapist is certified or licensed and seek recommendations from trusted sources.

Conclusion:

Massage therapy offers numerous benefits, including stress reduction, pain relief, improved circulation, and mental well-being. By incorporating massages into a wellness routine and exploring various massage techniques, individuals can experience the positive effects of relaxation, pain reduction, and overall improvement in physical and mental health.

CHAPTER 13

Understanding Dietary Changes for Back Pain Relief:

Why are Dietary Changes Important for Back Pain?

Making dietary adjustments can significantly impact inflammation levels, weight management, and overall health, potentially alleviating back pain.

Importance of Dietary Changes:

Reducing Inflammation: Certain foods can either increase or decrease inflammation levels in the body. Choosing anti-inflammatory foods may help reduce back pain caused by inflammation.

Weight Management: Maintaining a healthy weight through proper nutrition can reduce strain on the back, minimizing pressure on the spine and supporting overall back health.

Supporting Bone Health: Adequate intake of nutrients like calcium and vitamin D is essential for bone health, potentially reducing the risk of back problems such as osteoporosis.

Improving Overall Health: A balanced diet supports overall well-being, providing essential nutrients that aid in healing, tissue repair, and reducing the risk of chronic conditions related to back pain.

Dietary Tips for Back Pain Relief:

Anti-Inflammatory Foods:

Include foods rich in omega-3 fatty acids (salmon, chia seeds) and antioxidants (berries, leafy greens) to reduce inflammation.

Calcium and Vitamin D-Rich Foods:

Consume dairy products, leafy greens, nuts, and fortified cereals to support bone health.

Healthy Fats:

Incorporate sources of healthy fats like avocados, olive oil, and nuts to reduce inflammation and support overall health.

Hydration:

Stay adequately hydrated by drinking plenty of water to maintain spinal disc hydration and support overall health.

Limit Processed Foods and Sugars:

Reduce intake of processed foods, sugary snacks, and drinks to minimize inflammation and support weight management.

Incorporating Dietary Changes into Lifestyle:

Gradually introduce dietary changes to ensure sustainable habits.

Consult with a healthcare professional or nutritionist for personalized dietary advice tailored to back health.

Safety Precautions:

Ensure any drastic dietary changes align with personal health conditions or dietary restrictions.

Avoid extreme diets and seek balanced nutrition for long-term health benefits.

Conclusion:

Dietary changes play a crucial role in managing back pain by reducing inflammation, supporting weight management, and promoting overall health. By adopting a diet rich in anti-inflammatory foods, essential nutrients, and maintaining a healthy weight, individuals can potentially alleviate back pain and support better spinal health and overall well-being.

CHAPTER 14

Understanding the Importance of Seeking Professional Medical Advice:

Why is Seeking Medical Advice Important?

Consulting with healthcare professionals is crucial for accurate diagnosis, treatment, and guidance regarding health concerns, including back pain.

Importance of Seeking Professional Medical Advice:

Accurate Diagnosis: Healthcare professionals can accurately diagnose the underlying cause of back pain through physical examination, tests, and medical history assessment.

Tailored Treatment Plans: Based on the diagnosis, healthcare providers can develop personalized treatment plans, including medication, therapy, or referrals to specialists if needed.

Prevention of Complications: Early intervention and professional guidance can prevent back pain from worsening, reducing the risk of complications or chronic conditions.

Access to Specialized Care: Seeking medical advice allows access to specialized care and advanced treatments that may not be available through self-diagnosis or home remedies.

Patient Education: Healthcare professionals provide valuable information, educating patients about their condition, preventive measures, and lifestyle changes for better back health.

When to Seek Medical Advice:

Persistent Pain: If back pain persists for more than a few days despite self-care measures or worsens over time.

Severe Pain or New Symptoms: Severe pain, numbness, tingling, or weakness in the legs or feet warrant immediate medical attention.

History of Medical Conditions: Individuals with existing health conditions or previous back injuries should consult healthcare professionals for proper management.

Steps to Seeking Professional Medical Advice:

Primary Care Physician:

Start by consulting a primary care physician who can evaluate the condition and recommend further steps if necessary.

Specialists:

If needed, the primary care physician may refer to orthopedists, neurologists, or physical therapists for specialized care.

Diagnostic Tests:

Healthcare providers may conduct tests like X-rays, MRIs, or CT scans to identify the cause of back pain accurately.

Safety Precautions:

Be honest and thorough while discussing symptoms and medical history with healthcare providers.

Follow the advice and treatment plans prescribed by healthcare professionals for optimal results.

Conclusion:

Seeking professional medical advice is crucial for accurate diagnosis, personalized treatment plans, and preventive care for back pain. By consulting healthcare professionals promptly and following their guidance, individuals can receive appropriate care, manage back pain effectively, and prioritize their overall health and well-being.

CHAPTER 15

Understanding Over-the-Counter (OTC) Medications:

What are Over-the-Counter Medications?

Over-the-counter medications are drugs available without a prescription, easily accessible at pharmacies or stores for self-treatment of minor ailments.

Importance of Over-the-Counter Medications:

Managing Minor Ailments: OTC medications are suitable for treating common health issues like headaches, muscle aches, and minor back pain.

Convenience and Accessibility: Easily available without a doctor's prescription, providing quick relief for minor ailments.

Affordability: OTC medications are generally more affordable than prescription medications, making them accessible for most individuals.

Variety of Options: There are diverse OTC options tailored to various symptoms and conditions, providing choices for individuals' preferences.

Common Types of OTC Medications for Back Pain:

Pain Relievers (Analgesics):

Acetaminophen and Nonsteroidal Anti-Inflammatory Drugs (NSAIDs) like ibuprofen or naproxen sodium can help alleviate mild to moderate back pain.

Topical Treatments:

Creams, gels, or patches containing menthol, capsaicin, or lidocaine may provide localized relief when applied directly to the affected area.

Muscle Relaxants:

Some OTC muscle relaxants may help alleviate muscle spasms or tension contributing to back pain.

Using OTC Medications Safely:

Read Labels Carefully: Follow dosage instructions and warnings on the medication labels.

Consult a Healthcare Provider: Seek advice from a healthcare professional before using new medications, especially if pregnant, nursing, or have existing health conditions.

Avoid Long-Term Use: Limit the use of OTC medications for an extended period without consulting a healthcare provider.

When to Consult a Healthcare Professional:

If back pain persists or worsens despite using OTC medications.

If experiencing side effects or adverse reactions from OTC medications.

Safety Precautions:

Do not exceed recommended dosages to avoid potential side effects or complications.

Keep OTC medications out of reach of children and follow storage guidelines.

Conclusion:

Over-the-counter medications provide accessible and convenient relief for minor back pain and common ailments. While they offer benefits in managing mild symptoms, it's essential to use them responsibly by following dosage instructions, being aware of potential side effects, and seeking professional advice when necessary to ensure safe and effective use.

CHAPTER 16

Understanding the Role of Stress in Back Pain:

How Does Stress Affect Back Pain?

Stress can contribute to back pain by causing muscle tension, affecting posture, and increasing susceptibility to discomfort or injury.

Importance of Addressing Stress for Back Pain:

Muscle Tension: Stress triggers muscle tension, especially in the back and neck, leading to stiffness, discomfort, and increased risk of strains.

Postural Changes: Stress can influence posture, causing individuals to adopt positions that strain the back muscles, contributing to pain and discomfort.

Impact on Pain Perception: Emotional stress can heighten pain perception, making individuals more sensitive to back pain.

Chronic Back Pain: Prolonged stress can exacerbate existing back pain or contribute to the development of chronic back problems.

Managing Stress for Back Pain Relief:

Stress Reduction Techniques:

Engage in relaxation techniques such as deep breathing, meditation, or yoga to alleviate stress and muscle tension.

Physical Activity:

Regular exercise helps reduce stress levels, improves mood, and supports overall well-being, potentially reducing back pain.

Healthy Lifestyle:

Maintain a balanced diet, adequate sleep, and healthy lifestyle habits to better manage stress and its impact on back pain.

Seeking Support:

Talk to friends, family, or a healthcare professional for emotional support or guidance on stress management techniques.

Identifying Stress Triggers:

Recognize stressors in daily life, such as work pressure, personal relationships, or lifestyle factors, and develop strategies to manage them effectively.

Coping Strategies for Stress-Induced Back Pain:

Practice mindfulness and relaxation techniques to alleviate muscle tension and reduce stress-related discomfort.

Ensure a supportive work environment and practice ergonomic habits to reduce physical stress on the back during daily activities.

Seeking Professional Help:

If stress-related back pain persists or becomes chronic, seek guidance from healthcare professionals or mental health experts for specialized care or interventions.

Conclusion:

Stress plays a significant role in exacerbating back pain by causing muscle tension, affecting posture, and increasing pain perception. By employing stress management techniques, adopting healthy lifestyle habits, and seeking professional support when needed, individuals can effectively reduce stress levels, alleviate back pain, and promote overall well-being.

CHAPTER 17

Understanding Acupuncture and Acupressure:

What are Acupuncture and Acupressure?

Acupuncture and acupressure are ancient therapeutic practices originating from Traditional Chinese Medicine (TCM) that involve stimulating specific points on the body to alleviate pain and promote healing.

Importance of Acupuncture and Acupressure for Back Pain:

Pain Relief: Both acupuncture and acupressure are believed to help reduce back pain by promoting the body's natural pain-relieving mechanisms.

Improved Energy Flow: TCM principles suggest that these therapies help balance the flow of "qi" or vital energy along specific pathways called meridians, aiding in pain relief and overall well-being.

Muscle Relaxation: By targeting specific points, these therapies may help relax tense muscles contributing to back pain.

Stress Reduction: Acupuncture and acupressure may promote relaxation and reduce stress, potentially alleviating stress-related back pain.

Acupuncture vs. Acupressure:

Acupuncture: Involves inserting thin needles at specific points on the body to stimulate nerve endings, promoting pain relief and healing.

Acupressure: Utilizes finger pressure on specific points without needles, aiming to achieve similar benefits as acupuncture.

Potential Benefits:

Non-Invasive Nature: Both acupuncture and acupressure are generally considered safe and non-invasive methods for managing back pain.

Complementary Therapy: They can be used alongside conventional treatments to enhance pain relief and support overall well-being.

Customized Approach: Acupuncture and acupressure can be tailored to individual needs, focusing on specific points related to back pain.

Safety and Considerations:

Certified Practitioners: Ensure treatments are administered by certified and trained practitioners to ensure safety and effectiveness.

Consultation: Discuss any existing health conditions, allergies, or concerns with the practitioner before treatment.

Potential Mild Discomfort: Some individuals may experience slight discomfort or tingling during acupuncture sessions.

Conclusion:

Acupuncture and acupressure are alternative therapies that offer potential benefits in relieving back pain by targeting specific points on the body to promote healing and pain relief. When administered by certified practitioners and used alongside conventional treatments, these therapies may provide a non-invasive option for managing back pain and improving overall well-being.

CHAPTER 18

Understanding Chiropractic Care for Back Pain:

What is Chiropractic Care?

Chiropractic care is a healthcare approach that focuses on the diagnosis, treatment, and prevention of musculoskeletal disorders, including back pain, through manual adjustments and spinal manipulation.

Importance of Chiropractic Care for Back Pain:

Spinal Alignment: Chiropractors use manual adjustments to realign the spine, aiming to alleviate pressure on nerves, reduce inflammation, and improve mobility.

Pain Relief: Chiropractic adjustments can potentially reduce back pain by addressing misalignments or imbalances that contribute to discomfort.

Improving Function: By restoring spinal alignment, chiropractic care may enhance the body's natural healing abilities and functional performance.

Holistic Approach: Chiropractors often emphasize lifestyle modifications, exercises, and ergonomic advice to support long-term back health.

Chiropractic Techniques:

Spinal Manipulation: Manual adjustments involve controlled, sudden force applied to specific spinal joints to improve range of motion and alleviate pain.

Mobilization: Gentle stretching or movement of the spine to improve flexibility and reduce stiffness.

Soft Tissue Therapies: Additional treatments such as massage, electrical stimulation, or therapeutic exercises may complement spinal adjustments.

Potential Benefits:

Non-Invasive Approach: Chiropractic care offers a drug-free, non-surgical alternative for managing back pain.

Individualized Treatment: Chiropractors tailor treatment plans based on the patient's condition, considering their health history and specific needs.

Complementary Care: Chiropractic care can complement conventional medical treatments, enhancing overall back pain management.

Safety Considerations:

Certified Practitioners: Ensure treatment is administered by licensed and experienced chiropractors to ensure safety and effectiveness.

Pre-existing Conditions: Discuss any existing health conditions or concerns with the chiropractor before treatment.

Possible Mild Discomfort: Some individuals may experience temporary soreness or discomfort after adjustments, which typically subsides quickly.

Conclusion:

Chiropractic care offers a non-invasive approach to managing back pain by focusing on spinal alignment, improving function, and potentially reducing discomfort. When performed by certified practitioners and integrated with an individualized treatment plan, chiropractic care may provide an effective option for alleviating back pain and supporting overall spinal health.

CHAPTER 19

Understanding the Benefits of Physical Therapy:

What is Physical Therapy?

Physical therapy is a healthcare discipline focused on improving movement, relieving pain, and enhancing overall functionality through specialized exercises, manual techniques, and patient education.

Importance of Physical Therapy for Back Pain:

Pain Management: Physical therapists use targeted exercises and techniques to alleviate back pain, aiming to reduce discomfort and improve mobility.

Improved Function: Through customized treatment plans, physical therapy aims to restore strength, flexibility, and function in the affected areas of the back.

Preventing Recurrence: Physical therapy helps address underlying issues contributing to back pain, reducing the risk of future injuries or recurring pain.

Education and Self-Care: Patients receive guidance on proper posture, ergonomics, and exercises to manage back pain independently.

Components of Physical Therapy:

Exercise Programs: Tailored exercises to strengthen back muscles, improve flexibility, and enhance posture, reducing back pain.

Manual Therapy: Hands-on techniques such as massage, joint mobilization, or manipulation to alleviate pain and improve mobility.

Modalities: Application of heat, ice, ultrasound, or electrical stimulation to reduce pain and promote healing.

Education and Prevention: Guidance on proper body mechanics, posture, and lifestyle modifications to prevent future back issues.

Potential Benefits:

Non-Invasive Approach: Physical therapy offers non-surgical and drug-free methods for managing back pain.

Individualized Treatment: Therapists customize treatment plans according to each patient's specific needs and goals.

Functional Improvement: Physical therapy helps patients regain functional abilities necessary for daily activities.

Safety Considerations:

Qualified Practitioners: Seek treatment from licensed physical therapists with appropriate qualifications and certifications.

Communication: Discuss any concerns, allergies, or pre-existing conditions with the therapist to ensure safe and effective treatment.

Conclusion:

Physical therapy plays a vital role in managing back pain by focusing on pain relief, improving function, and preventing recurrence. Through personalized treatment plans comprising exercises, manual techniques, and patient education, physical therapy offers a non-invasive approach to alleviate back pain, restore functionality, and support overall back health.

CHAPTER 20

Understanding Lumbar Support Pillows/Cushions:

What are Lumbar Support Pillows?

Lumbar support pillows or cushions are specially designed cushions that provide additional support to the lower back (lumbar region) while sitting or lying down.

Importance of Lumbar Support for Back Health:

Maintaining Proper Posture: Lumbar support cushions help maintain the natural curvature of the spine while sitting, reducing strain on the lower back.

Alleviating Pressure: They provide additional support to the lower back, reducing pressure on the spine, and potentially alleviating back pain.

Improving Comfort: Lumbar cushions enhance seating comfort by promoting better posture and reducing discomfort during prolonged sitting.

Types of Lumbar Support Cushions:

Contoured Pillows: Ergonomically designed cushions with curves to fit the natural shape of the lower back.

Adjustable Cushions: Pillows with straps or adjustable features allowing customization for different chairs or body types.

Memory Foam or Gel Cushions: Pillows made from memory foam or gel that conform to the shape of the lower back, providing personalized support.

Benefits of Using Lumbar Support:

Posture Improvement: By supporting the natural spinal curve, these cushions aid in maintaining proper posture, reducing strain on the back muscles.

Pain Relief: Lumbar support cushions may alleviate discomfort and reduce the intensity of back pain by providing targeted support.

Versatility: They can be used in various settings, including office chairs, car seats, or even at home, offering consistent back support.

Using Lumbar Support Cushions:

Positioning: Place the cushion against the lower back region while seated, ensuring it supports the natural curve of the spine.

Regular Use: Consistently using the lumbar support cushion, especially during prolonged sitting, can maximize its benefits.

Safety Considerations:

Choosing the Right Cushion: Select a cushion that suits individual needs and preferences, considering factors like firmness and size.

Consultation: If experiencing severe or persistent back pain, consult a healthcare professional for appropriate guidance.

Conclusion:

Lumbar support pillows or cushions are valuable aids in promoting better posture, reducing strain on the lower back, and potentially alleviating back pain during prolonged sitting. By providing targeted support to the lumbar region, these cushions offer a simple and effective way to enhance seating comfort and support overall back health.

CHAPTER 21

Understanding Yoga and Its Impact on Back Health:

What is Yoga?

Yoga is a mind-body practice involving physical postures, breathing exercises, and meditation aimed at promoting holistic health and well-being.

Importance of Yoga for Back Health:

Improved Flexibility: Yoga poses (asanas) help stretch and lengthen muscles, increasing flexibility and reducing stiffness in the back.

Strengthening Core Muscles: Engaging in yoga strengthens the core muscles, including those supporting the spine, leading to better posture and reduced back strain.

Enhanced Posture Awareness: Yoga encourages body awareness, teaching individuals to maintain proper alignment and posture, which can alleviate back pain.

Stress Reduction: Breathing techniques and mindfulness practiced in yoga can reduce stress levels, potentially relieving stress-related back pain.

Yoga Poses Beneficial for Back Health:

Cat-Cow Stretch: Alternating between arching and rounding the back to increase spinal flexibility.

Child's Pose: A resting posture that gently stretches the lower back muscles.

Downward-Facing Dog: Stretches the entire spine and helps lengthen the back muscles.

Cobra Pose: Strengthens back muscles and opens the chest, promoting spinal flexibility.

Benefits of Practicing Yoga:

Pain Relief: Regular yoga practice may alleviate back pain by improving flexibility, strength, and posture.

Stress Reduction: Mindfulness and relaxation techniques in yoga can reduce stress, potentially easing tension-related back discomfort.

Enhanced Well-being: Yoga offers mental clarity, relaxation, and improved overall physical health, contributing to better back health.

Precautions and Safety Tips:

Guidance from Instructors: Beginners should seek guidance from certified yoga instructors to ensure proper techniques and prevent injury.

Modify Poses: Individuals with existing back conditions should modify poses or avoid certain movements to prevent exacerbating pain.

Gradual Progression: Start with gentle poses and gradually progress to more challenging ones to avoid strain or injury.

Conclusion:

Yoga is a beneficial practice for improving back health by enhancing flexibility, strengthening core muscles, and promoting better posture. Through regular practice and guidance from certified instructors, individuals can experience reduced back pain, improved flexibility, and overall well-being, making yoga a valuable tool in supporting back health.

CHAPTER 22

Understanding Pilates Exercises for Core Strength:

What is Pilates?

Pilates is a form of exercise that focuses on building strength, flexibility, and endurance using controlled movements primarily targeting the core muscles.

Importance of Pilates for Core Strength:

Core Muscle Engagement: Pilates emphasizes strengthening the core muscles, including the abdomen, lower back, hips, and pelvis, essential for supporting the spine.

Improved Posture: By strengthening the core, Pilates helps improve posture, reducing strain on the back and promoting better alignment.

Enhanced Stability: Pilates exercises aim to improve stability and balance by engaging core muscles, reducing the risk of back injuries.

Flexibility and Range of Motion: Pilates incorporates stretching movements that improve flexibility, reducing muscle tension contributing to back discomfort.

Pilates Exercises Beneficial for Core Strength:

The Hundred: Involves breathing while engaging the abdominal muscles, promoting core stability and endurance.

Leg Circle Exercise: Engages core muscles while moving the legs in circular motions, enhancing hip and pelvic stability.

Rolling Like a Ball: Strengthens the core by rolling on the back, engaging abdominal muscles for stability.

Plank Variations: Various plank exercises strengthen the core muscles, improving overall stability and reducing back strain.

Benefits of Practicing Pilates:

Core Strengthening: Pilates focuses on strengthening core muscles, which provides stability and support to the spine, reducing back strain.

Improved Posture: Engaging core muscles in Pilates exercises promotes better alignment, reducing the risk of back pain associated with poor posture.

Enhanced Flexibility: Pilates incorporates stretching movements that improve flexibility, reducing muscle tension contributing to back discomfort.

Mind-Body Connection: Pilates emphasizes concentration and mindful movements, promoting awareness of body alignment and posture.

Precautions and Safety Tips:

Professional Guidance: Beginners should seek guidance from certified Pilates instructors to ensure proper techniques and prevent injury.

Start Slowly: Begin with simple Pilates exercises and gradually progress to more advanced movements to avoid strain.

Listen to the Body: Individuals with existing back conditions should avoid movements causing discomfort and modify exercises accordingly.

Conclusion:

Pilates exercises are an effective way to strengthen core muscles, improve posture, and promote overall back health. Through regular practice, guided by certified instructors, individuals can experience enhanced core strength, reduced back strain, and improved stability, making Pilates a valuable tool in supporting back health.

CHAPTER 23

Understanding Hydrotherapy and Water-Based Exercises:

What is Hydrotherapy?

Hydrotherapy involves the use of water for therapeutic purposes, including exercises performed in water to improve health and well-being.

Importance of Hydrotherapy for Back Health:

Buoyancy Support: Water reduces the impact on joints, providing support while exercising and reducing strain on the back.

Muscle Relaxation: Immersion in warm water can help relax muscles, alleviating tension and potentially reducing back pain.

Increased Range of Motion: Water-based exercises promote movement in various directions, improving flexibility and range of motion in the back.

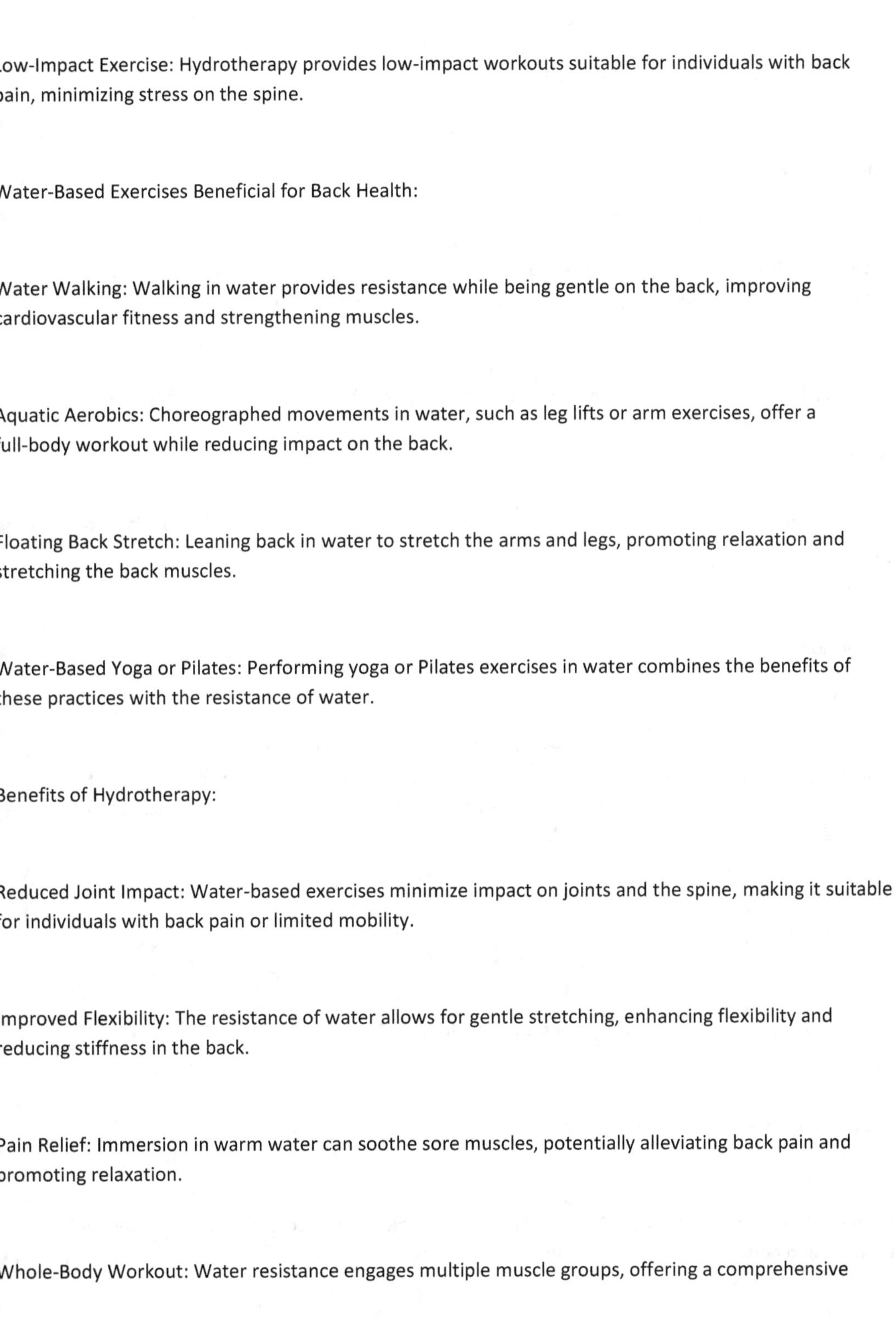

Low-Impact Exercise: Hydrotherapy provides low-impact workouts suitable for individuals with back pain, minimizing stress on the spine.

Water-Based Exercises Beneficial for Back Health:

Water Walking: Walking in water provides resistance while being gentle on the back, improving cardiovascular fitness and strengthening muscles.

Aquatic Aerobics: Choreographed movements in water, such as leg lifts or arm exercises, offer a full-body workout while reducing impact on the back.

Floating Back Stretch: Leaning back in water to stretch the arms and legs, promoting relaxation and stretching the back muscles.

Water-Based Yoga or Pilates: Performing yoga or Pilates exercises in water combines the benefits of these practices with the resistance of water.

Benefits of Hydrotherapy:

Reduced Joint Impact: Water-based exercises minimize impact on joints and the spine, making it suitable for individuals with back pain or limited mobility.

Improved Flexibility: The resistance of water allows for gentle stretching, enhancing flexibility and reducing stiffness in the back.

Pain Relief: Immersion in warm water can soothe sore muscles, potentially alleviating back pain and promoting relaxation.

Whole-Body Workout: Water resistance engages multiple muscle groups, offering a comprehensive workout while targeting the back muscles.

Safety and Considerations:

Supervision: Perform water exercises under the supervision of a trained professional, especially if unfamiliar with swimming or aquatic workouts.

Gradual Progression: Start with gentle movements and gradually increase intensity or duration to prevent overexertion.

Consultation: Individuals with medical conditions should consult healthcare professionals before starting hydrotherapy exercises.

Conclusion:

Hydrotherapy and water-based exercises provide a low-impact, therapeutic approach to improve back health. By offering support, reducing strain, and promoting relaxation, these exercises can enhance flexibility, reduce back pain, and improve overall well-being, making them a valuable option in supporting back health for many individuals.

CHAPTER 24

Understanding Cognitive Behavioral Therapy (CBT) for Pain Management:

What is Cognitive Behavioral Therapy?

Cognitive Behavioral Therapy (CBT) is a form of psychotherapy that focuses on changing thought patterns and behaviors to manage emotions and improve well-being.

Importance of CBT for Pain Management:

Changing Perception: CBT helps individuals reframe thoughts about pain, altering the perception of pain and its impact on daily life.

Behavioral Techniques: Teaches coping strategies and behavioral techniques to manage pain and improve overall functioning.

Addressing Emotional Impact: CBT addresses emotions related to pain, such as anxiety or depression, which can exacerbate discomfort.

Enhancing Coping Skills: Encourages the development of effective coping skills to handle pain, reducing its impact on daily activities.

Components of CBT for Pain Management:

Cognitive Restructuring: Identifies and challenges negative thought patterns related to pain, replacing them with more balanced thoughts.

Behavioral Activation: Encourages engaging in enjoyable activities and increasing physical movement, despite pain, to improve mood and function.

Relaxation Techniques: Teaches relaxation methods such as deep breathing or progressive muscle relaxation to reduce tension and pain perception.

Pain Coping Skills: Provides skills to manage pain, including distraction techniques or guided imagery, to redirect focus away from discomfort.

Benefits of CBT for Pain Management:

Improved Pain Coping Strategies: CBT equips individuals with practical tools to manage pain and minimize its interference in daily life.

Enhanced Functionality: By addressing thoughts and behaviors around pain, CBT helps individuals regain function and engage in meaningful activities.

Reduced Emotional Impact: CBT assists in managing emotional distress related to pain, such as anxiety or depression, improving overall well-being.

Long-term Effectiveness: Research suggests that CBT can lead to lasting improvements in pain management even after therapy concludes.

Safety and Considerations:

Professional Guidance: CBT should be conducted by trained therapists specializing in pain management.

Commitment to Practice: Consistent practice of CBT techniques is essential for achieving beneficial outcomes.

Individual Tailoring: Therapy should be customized to address each individual's specific pain experience and needs.

Conclusion:

Cognitive Behavioral Therapy offers a structured approach to pain management by addressing thought patterns, emotions, and behaviors related to pain. Through the development of coping skills, changing perceptions, and enhancing functionality, CBT can empower individuals to better manage pain, improve daily functioning, and enhance overall well-being, making it a valuable tool in pain management strategies.

CHAPTER 25

Understanding Supportive Shoe Choices and Footwear:

Importance of Supportive Footwear:

Supportive footwear plays a crucial role in providing comfort, stability, and reducing strain on the feet, ultimately benefiting overall posture and body alignment.

Features of Supportive Footwear:

Arch Support: Shoes with adequate arch support help distribute weight evenly, reducing stress on the arches and minimizing discomfort.

Cushioning: Quality cushioning absorbs impact, providing shock absorption and reducing strain on the feet and lower limbs.

Proper Fit: Well-fitted shoes with ample room for toes and a snug fit around the heel prevent issues like blisters and ensure comfort during movement.

Sturdy Soles: Shoes with firm, supportive soles offer stability, reducing the risk of tripping or twisting ankles.

Types of Supportive Footwear:

Orthopedic Shoes: Specifically designed to address foot conditions, providing extra support and comfort for individuals with foot problems.

Athletic Shoes: Many brands offer sports shoes designed with cushioning, support, and stability for various activities, benefiting overall foot health.

Comfort Shoes: Casual footwear designed for everyday wear, often with additional features such as cushioned insoles and arch support.

Benefits of Supportive Footwear:

Reduced Foot Pain: Supportive shoes can alleviate foot pain by providing better arch support and cushioning impact while walking or standing.

Improved Posture: Properly fitted shoes contribute to better posture, reducing strain on the feet, ankles, knees, and lower back.

Enhanced Stability: Shoes with supportive soles offer stability, reducing the risk of slips or falls, especially in uneven terrain.

Prevention of Foot Problems: Good footwear choices can prevent common foot issues like plantar fasciitis, bunions, or corns.

Selecting Supportive Footwear:

Try Before Buying: Test shoes for comfort and fit, ensuring they feel supportive and don't cause any discomfort.

Consider Foot Type: Choose shoes based on individual foot type and any specific foot conditions or concerns.

Replace When Worn: Regularly replace worn-out shoes to maintain adequate support and cushioning.

Conclusion:

Supportive footwear with features like proper arch support, cushioning, and a good fit plays a vital role in maintaining foot health, reducing discomfort, and promoting better posture. By selecting footwear that prioritizes support and comfort, individuals can alleviate foot pain, enhance stability, and prevent various foot-related problems, contributing to overall well-being and comfort in daily activities.

CHAPTER 26

Understanding the Role of Inflammation in Back Pain:

What is Inflammation?

Inflammation is the body's natural response to injury, infection, or irritation, involving the immune system's protective response to remove harmful stimuli and initiate the healing process.

How Inflammation Affects Back Pain:

Source of Pain: Inflammation can be a source of pain in various back conditions, such as sciatica, arthritis, or muscle strain.

Nerve Irritation: Inflammatory responses near nerves in the back can cause irritation or compression, leading to pain signals sent to the brain.

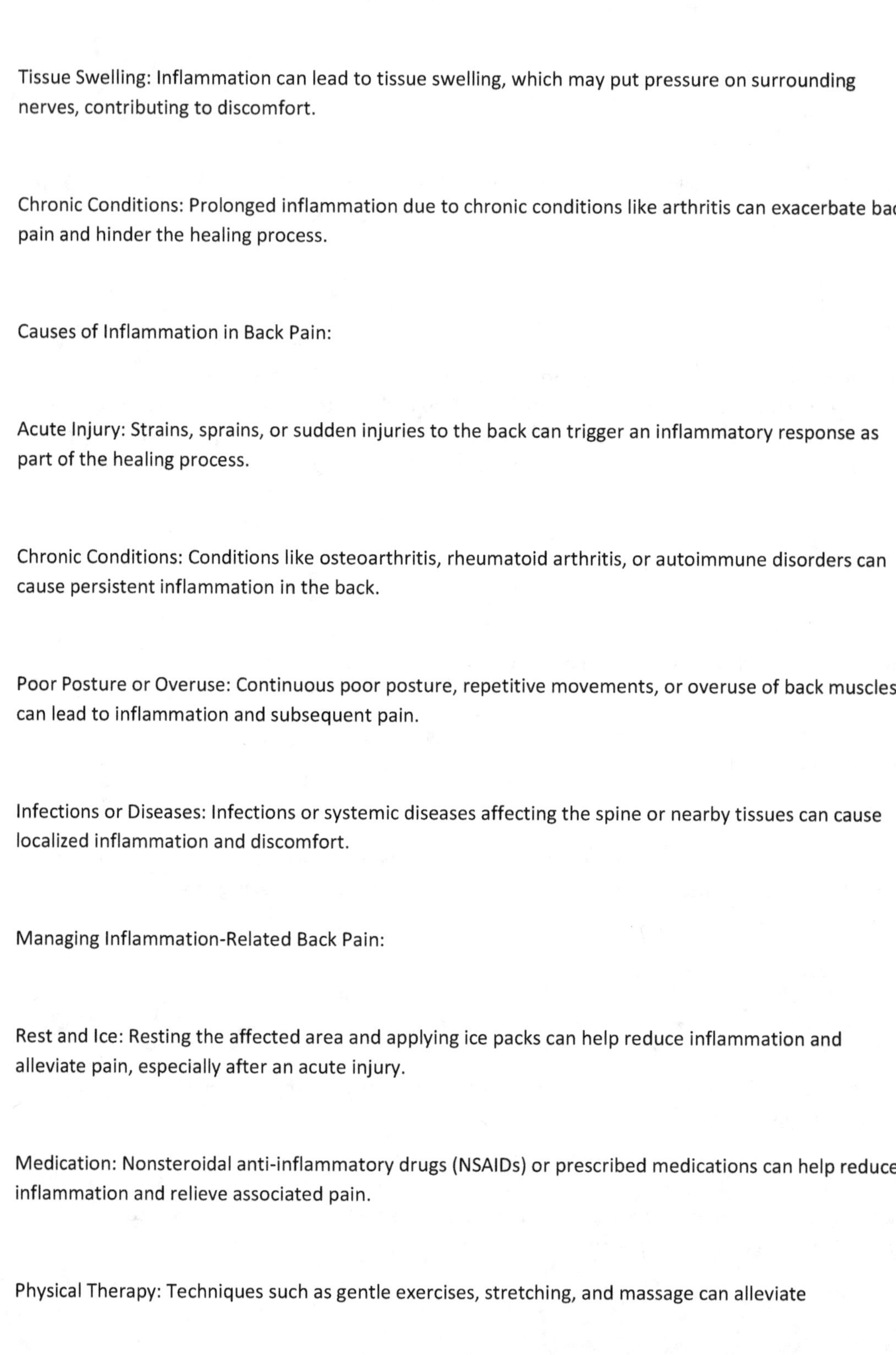

Tissue Swelling: Inflammation can lead to tissue swelling, which may put pressure on surrounding nerves, contributing to discomfort.

Chronic Conditions: Prolonged inflammation due to chronic conditions like arthritis can exacerbate back pain and hinder the healing process.

Causes of Inflammation in Back Pain:

Acute Injury: Strains, sprains, or sudden injuries to the back can trigger an inflammatory response as part of the healing process.

Chronic Conditions: Conditions like osteoarthritis, rheumatoid arthritis, or autoimmune disorders can cause persistent inflammation in the back.

Poor Posture or Overuse: Continuous poor posture, repetitive movements, or overuse of back muscles can lead to inflammation and subsequent pain.

Infections or Diseases: Infections or systemic diseases affecting the spine or nearby tissues can cause localized inflammation and discomfort.

Managing Inflammation-Related Back Pain:

Rest and Ice: Resting the affected area and applying ice packs can help reduce inflammation and alleviate pain, especially after an acute injury.

Medication: Nonsteroidal anti-inflammatory drugs (NSAIDs) or prescribed medications can help reduce inflammation and relieve associated pain.

Physical Therapy: Techniques such as gentle exercises, stretching, and massage can alleviate inflammation-related discomfort.

Healthy Lifestyle: Maintaining a healthy weight, regular exercise, and a balanced diet can help reduce inflammation in chronic back conditions.

Seeking Medical Attention:

Persistent Pain: If back pain persists or worsens despite home remedies, it's crucial to consult a healthcare professional for proper diagnosis and treatment.

New Symptoms: Any new symptoms like numbness, tingling, weakness, or fever alongside back pain should be evaluated by a medical professional.

Conclusion:

Inflammation plays a significant role in back pain, whether due to acute injuries, chronic conditions, or other underlying issues. Understanding the link between inflammation and back discomfort helps individuals implement appropriate strategies such as rest, medication, therapy, and healthy lifestyle choices to manage inflammation-related back pain effectively. Seeking medical advice for persistent or worsening symptoms is essential to address inflammation-related issues and promote back health.

CHAPTER 27

Understanding Workplace Ergonomics and Back Health:

What is Workplace Ergonomics?

Workplace ergonomics focuses on designing the work environment to fit the needs of the individual, aiming to optimize comfort, efficiency, and reduce the risk of musculoskeletal issues like back pain.

Importance of Workplace Ergonomics for Back Health:

Posture Support: Proper ergonomic setups promote good posture, reducing strain on the back and minimizing discomfort.

Reduced Strain: Ergonomic adjustments in workstations help alleviate stress on the back muscles and spine, preventing long-term issues.

Improved Comfort: Well-designed work environments enhance comfort, reducing the likelihood of back-related discomfort during work hours.

Enhanced Productivity: Ergonomic setups ensure workers are comfortable and less prone to discomfort, promoting focus and productivity.

Ergonomic Factors Impacting Back Health:

Proper Desk Setup: Adjusting desk height, chair positioning, and monitor height to maintain neutral spine posture while seated.

Chair Support: Using chairs with lumbar support to maintain the natural curve of the spine and reduce strain on the lower back.

Keyboard and Mouse Placement: Placing these devices at an ergonomic level to prevent reaching or straining the arms and shoulders.

Regular Breaks and Movement: Encouraging short breaks and movement to reduce prolonged sitting, allowing muscles to relax and preventing stiffness.

Benefits of Workplace Ergonomics for Back Health:

Reduced Back Pain: Properly designed workstations reduce strain on the back, minimizing discomfort and the risk of developing back-related issues.

Improved Posture: Ergonomic setups encourage correct posture, supporting the spine's natural alignment and reducing back strain.

Enhanced Comfort: Adjustments in workstations improve overall comfort, allowing employees to focus better on their tasks without experiencing discomfort.

Prevention of Injuries: Ergonomically designed workplaces lower the risk of repetitive strain injuries and musculoskeletal issues associated with poor ergonomics.

Implementing Ergonomic Practices:

Workstation Assessment: Employers should conduct assessments to ensure workstations are ergonomically suitable for employees.

Training and Education: Educating employees about proper ergonomics and encouraging correct postures and practices at work.

Adjustments and Support: Employers should provide adjustable chairs, supportive equipment, and resources for employees to create ergonomic workspaces.

Conclusion:

Workplace ergonomics plays a vital role in promoting back health by providing ergonomic setups that support good posture, reduce strain on the back, and enhance overall comfort. By implementing ergonomic practices and providing proper support and education, employers can create work environments that minimize the risk of back-related discomfort or injuries, allowing employees to work comfortably and productively while maintaining their back health.

CHAPTER 28

Understanding Mindfulness and Meditation Practices:

What is Mindfulness?

Mindfulness involves being fully present and aware of one's thoughts, feelings, bodily sensations, and the surrounding environment without judgment.

What is Meditation?

Meditation refers to a variety of techniques that encourage relaxation, focus, and awareness to achieve a calm and tranquil state of mind.

Importance of Mindfulness and Meditation:

Stress Reduction: Mindfulness and meditation help reduce stress by promoting relaxation and enhancing self-awareness.

Improved Mental Well-being: These practices can improve mental clarity, focus, and emotional regulation, leading to a sense of calmness.

Enhanced Physical Health: Studies suggest that regular meditation practices may reduce blood pressure, improve sleep, and alleviate chronic pain.

Better Coping Skills: Mindfulness and meditation cultivate coping mechanisms, allowing individuals to respond more effectively to life's challenges.

Types of Mindfulness and Meditation Practices:

Breath Awareness: Focusing on the breath, observing inhalation and exhalation to anchor attention and promote relaxation.

Body Scan: Scanning the body to notice sensations and tensions, gradually relaxing muscles and fostering body awareness.

Guided Meditation: Listening to guided instructions or recordings to facilitate relaxation and focus on specific thoughts or sensations.

Mindful Movement: Engaging in activities like walking or yoga with a heightened awareness of body movements and sensations.

Benefits of Mindfulness and Meditation:

Stress Reduction: Regular practice helps reduce stress by calming the mind and promoting a sense of relaxation.

Improved Focus: Enhances concentration and attention, allowing individuals to stay present and focused on tasks.

Emotional Regulation: Helps manage emotions by developing a greater understanding and acceptance of thoughts and feelings.

Better Sleep Quality: Promotes relaxation and reduces anxiety, potentially improving sleep patterns and quality.

Incorporating Mindfulness and Meditation:

Start Small: Begin with short sessions, gradually increasing duration as comfort and practice grow.

Consistency: Regular practice, even for a few minutes a day, can yield significant benefits over time.

Find a Comfortable Space: Choose a quiet, comfortable spot to practice without distractions.

Conclusion:

Mindfulness and meditation practices offer numerous benefits, including stress reduction, improved mental well-being, enhanced focus, and better coping skills. By incorporating these simple techniques into daily life, individuals can experience increased relaxation, emotional balance, and a greater sense of overall well-being, making mindfulness and meditation valuable tools for promoting mental and physical health.

CHAPTER 29

Understanding Tai Chi for Balance and Flexibility:

What is Tai Chi?

Tai Chi is a gentle form of exercise originating from China, characterized by slow, deliberate movements and deep breathing.

Importance of Tai Chi for Balance and Flexibility:

Enhanced Balance: Tai Chi involves controlled movements that help improve balance, reducing the risk of falls, especially in older adults.

Increased Flexibility: Gentle stretching and flowing motions in Tai Chi exercises enhance flexibility in muscles and joints.

Improved Coordination: Tai Chi movements promote body awareness and coordination, enhancing overall physical control.

Relaxation and Stress Reduction: The meditative nature of Tai Chi helps relax the mind and body, reducing stress and tension.

Tai Chi Techniques for Balance and Flexibility:

Slow, Fluid Movements: Tai Chi involves slow and continuous movements, promoting body awareness and flexibility.

Weight Shifting: Practitioners shift weight from one leg to another, improving stability and balance.

Deep Breathing: Controlled breathing techniques used in Tai Chi enhance relaxation and focus.

Mindful Meditation: Incorporating meditation practices while performing Tai Chi helps improve mental clarity and relaxation.

Benefits of Tai Chi for Balance and Flexibility:

Reduced Risk of Falls: Tai Chi exercises strengthen muscles and improve balance, reducing the risk of falls, especially in older adults.

Enhanced Flexibility: The gentle, flowing motions in Tai Chi promote joint mobility and flexibility.

Better Posture: Practicing Tai Chi encourages proper body alignment and posture, reducing strain on muscles and joints.

Stress Relief: Tai Chi's meditative aspects promote relaxation and stress reduction, benefiting both physical and mental well-being.

Incorporating Tai Chi:

Classes and Instruction: Joining Tai Chi classes or seeking instruction from a certified instructor to learn proper techniques.

Start Slow: Begin with basic movements and gradually progress as comfort and familiarity with the practice grow.

Consistency: Regular practice of Tai Chi yields better results in improving balance and flexibility.

Conclusion:

Tai Chi, with its slow, flowing movements and meditative qualities, offers numerous benefits for improving balance, flexibility, and overall well-being. By incorporating Tai Chi into a regular exercise routine, individuals can experience enhanced balance, increased flexibility, reduced stress, and improved coordination, making it a valuable practice for promoting physical and mental health.

CHAPTER 30

Understanding Posture Correcting Devices and Tools:

What are Posture Correcting Devices?

Posture correcting devices are tools or equipment designed to help improve body alignment, support the spine, and promote better posture.

Importance of Posture Correction:

Spinal Alignment: Proper posture reduces strain on the spine, supporting its natural alignment and minimizing discomfort.

Muscle Support: Posture correcting devices provide support to muscles, reducing fatigue and tension in the back and neck.

Enhanced Breathing: Improved posture allows for better lung expansion, facilitating easier breathing and reducing fatigue.

Prevention of Aches: Maintaining good posture can prevent aches and pains associated with poor alignment and strain on muscles.

Types of Posture Correcting Devices:

Posture Correctors: Devices worn around the shoulders or back to encourage proper alignment and support.

Ergonomic Chairs: Chairs designed with lumbar support to maintain the natural curve of the spine and improve seated posture.

Standing Desks: Height-adjustable desks that allow individuals to alternate between sitting and standing, promoting better posture.

Back Braces or Belts: Supportive belts or braces that offer back support and encourage proper spinal alignment.

Benefits of Posture Correcting Devices:

Improved Posture: These tools help train the body for better posture by providing support and reminding individuals to sit or stand properly.

Reduced Pain: Posture correcting devices alleviate strain on muscles and joints, reducing discomfort and preventing future pain.

Increased Awareness: Continuous use of these tools raises awareness about posture habits, encouraging mindful adjustments.

Enhanced Comfort: Properly designed devices offer comfort and support, allowing individuals to maintain better posture without strain.

Incorporating Posture Correcting Tools:

Proper Use: Follow instructions for wearing or using these devices correctly to achieve optimal benefits.

Gradual Progress: Begin using these tools gradually, allowing the body to adapt and adjust to improved posture.

Consistency: Regular use of posture correcting devices is essential for long-term benefits in correcting posture.

Conclusion:

Posture correcting devices and tools are valuable aids in improving body alignment, reducing strain on muscles, and preventing discomfort associated with poor posture. By incorporating these tools into daily routines, individuals can experience enhanced posture, reduced pain, and increased comfort, promoting overall well-being and supporting a healthier lifestyle.

CHAPTER 31

Understanding Avoidance of Prolonged Sitting:

What is Prolonged Sitting?

Prolonged sitting refers to extended periods of sitting or remaining sedentary without breaks for movement or activity.

Importance of Avoiding Prolonged Sitting:

Muscle Stiffness: Prolonged sitting can cause stiffness in muscles, especially in the back, hips, and legs.

Reduced Blood Flow: Long periods of sitting can decrease blood flow and circulation, leading to potential health risks.

Back Discomfort: Sitting for extended periods without breaks can strain the back and contribute to discomfort or pain.

Impact on Posture: Prolonged sitting may lead to poor posture, affecting spine alignment and muscle health.

Tips for Avoiding Prolonged Sitting:

Regular Breaks: Take short breaks every 30-60 minutes to stand up, stretch, or walk around, promoting blood circulation and reducing muscle stiffness.

Standing Desks: Use standing desks or adjustable desks that allow alternating between sitting and standing positions.

Movement Breaks: Incorporate short movements or exercises into the routine, like stretching, walking, or simple exercises to break up long periods of sitting.

Active Breaks: Engage in brief physical activities or chores during breaks, encouraging movement and reducing sedentary time.

Benefits of Avoiding Prolonged Sitting:

Improved Circulation: Frequent movement helps maintain blood flow, reducing the risk of blood clots and related health issues.

Reduced Muscle Stiffness: Regular breaks prevent muscle stiffness and tension, promoting comfort and flexibility.

Enhanced Energy Levels: Short movement breaks boost energy levels and productivity, preventing fatigue from prolonged sitting.

Better Posture: Alternating between sitting and standing promotes better posture, reducing strain on the back and improving spine alignment.

Incorporating Strategies to Avoid Prolonged Sitting:

Set Reminders: Use alarms or reminders to prompt breaks and movement every hour.

Create Opportunities: Find opportunities to stand or move during tasks, such as taking phone calls while standing or walking.

Mindful Awareness: Be mindful of sitting habits and consciously make efforts to break up extended periods of sitting.

Conclusion:

Avoiding prolonged sitting is crucial for maintaining overall health and reducing the risks associated with sedentary behavior. By incorporating regular breaks, movement, and standing activities into daily routines, individuals can combat the negative effects of prolonged sitting, promoting better circulation, muscle flexibility, and overall well-being.

CHAPTER 32

Understanding the Impact of Smoking on Back Pain:

Smoking and Back Pain:

Smoking can have detrimental effects on overall health, including its impact on back pain.

How Smoking Affects Back Pain:

Reduced Blood Flow: Smoking narrows blood vessels, reducing blood flow to spinal discs and muscles, hindering their ability to heal properly.

Disc Degeneration: Smoking can accelerate disc degeneration by depriving spinal discs of essential nutrients, contributing to back pain and stiffness.

Delayed Healing: Smokers tend to experience slower healing from back injuries due to reduced blood flow and impaired tissue repair.

Increased Pain Sensitivity: Smoking may increase pain sensitivity, making individuals more susceptible to experiencing back pain.

Connection Between Smoking and Back Pain:

Disc Degeneration: Smoking is associated with premature disc degeneration, leading to increased susceptibility to back pain.

Chronic Pain: Smokers are more likely to experience chronic back pain compared to non-smokers due to the adverse effects on spinal health.

Delayed Recovery: Individuals who smoke often experience delayed recovery from back injuries or surgeries due to compromised healing.

Impact on Treatment: Smoking can reduce the effectiveness of treatments for back pain, hindering the body's ability to respond to therapies.

Benefits of Quitting Smoking for Back Pain:

Improved Healing: Quitting smoking can enhance blood flow and nutrient delivery to the spine, aiding in the healing of injured tissues.

Reduced Degeneration: Ceasing smoking may slow down or prevent further degeneration of spinal discs, reducing the risk of chronic back pain.

Enhanced Treatment Response: Non-smokers tend to respond better to back pain treatments, enhancing the effectiveness of therapies.

Decreased Pain Sensitivity: Quitting smoking may lower pain sensitivity, leading to reduced back pain perception.

Taking Steps for Better Back Health:

Quitting Smoking: Seek support and resources to quit smoking, promoting better spinal health and reducing back pain risks.

Healthy Lifestyle: Engage in regular exercise, maintain a balanced diet, and practice good posture to support back health.

Seeking Help: Consult healthcare professionals for guidance on managing back pain and quitting smoking.

Conclusion:

Smoking can exacerbate back pain and hinder the body's ability to heal from injuries or degenerative conditions affecting the spine. Quitting smoking plays a significant role in improving spinal health, promoting better healing, reducing the risk of chronic back pain, and enhancing the effectiveness of back pain treatments. Embracing a smoke-free lifestyle is essential for supporting overall back health and minimizing the impact of smoking-related complications on back pain.

CHAPTER 33

Understanding Alternative Medicine Approaches:

What is Alternative Medicine?

Alternative medicine refers to a broad range of therapies and practices used in place of conventional medical treatments to promote healing and well-being.

Types of Alternative Medicine Approaches:

Acupuncture: Involves inserting thin needles into specific points on the body to alleviate pain and promote healing.

Chiropractic Care: Focuses on spinal manipulation and adjustments to treat musculoskeletal issues, including back pain.

Herbal Remedies: Uses plants and herbs for medicinal purposes, often in the form of supplements, teas, or extracts.

Massage Therapy: Involves manipulation of muscles and tissues to reduce muscle tension, improve circulation, and alleviate pain.

Mind-Body Techniques: Includes practices like yoga, tai chi, and meditation that promote relaxation, reduce stress, and improve overall well-being.

Benefits of Exploring Alternative Medicine Approaches:

Holistic Approach: Alternative medicine often takes a holistic approach, considering the whole person and focusing on overall health and well-being.

Natural Healing: Many alternative therapies use natural remedies and techniques to promote healing and alleviate symptoms.

Complementary Treatments: Some alternative therapies can complement conventional medical treatments to enhance their effectiveness.

Personalized Care: Alternative medicine often involves personalized treatments tailored to an individual's specific needs and preferences.

Effectiveness of Alternative Medicine Approaches for Back Pain:

Acupuncture: Studies suggest acupuncture may offer relief from chronic back pain by stimulating nerves and releasing endorphins.

Chiropractic Care: Chiropractic adjustments may improve spinal alignment, reduce pain, and enhance mobility in some back pain cases.

Herbal Remedies: Certain herbs like turmeric, ginger, or devil's claw may have anti-inflammatory properties that can ease back pain.

Massage Therapy: Regular massages can help relax muscles, reduce tension, and alleviate back pain symptoms.

Incorporating Alternative Medicine Approaches:

Consultation: Seek guidance from qualified practitioners or healthcare professionals before trying alternative therapies.

Open Communication: Discuss intentions to explore alternative treatments with primary healthcare providers for advice and coordination.

Trial and Observation: Give alternative treatments a fair trial while observing their effects on back pain and overall well-being.

Conclusion:

Alternative medicine approaches offer diverse methods that focus on natural healing, holistic care, and personalized treatments for various health conditions, including back pain. When exploring alternative therapies, it's crucial to do so under the guidance of qualified practitioners and in conjunction with conventional medical advice. While these approaches may offer benefits and relief for some individuals experiencing back pain, it's essential to approach them with an open mind and awareness of their potential role as complementary to conventional medical care.

CHAPTER 34

Understanding Chronic Back Pain Management:

What is Chronic Back Pain?

Chronic back pain refers to persistent discomfort or pain in the back that lasts for an extended period, typically more than 12 weeks.

Chronic Back Pain Management Strategies:

Physical Activity: Engage in low-impact exercises like walking, swimming, or yoga to strengthen muscles, improve flexibility, and reduce pain.

Posture Improvement: Practice proper posture while sitting, standing, and lifting to reduce strain on the back and maintain spinal alignment.

Hot and Cold Therapy: Apply heat or cold packs to the affected area to alleviate muscle spasms, reduce inflammation, and relieve pain.

Medications: Over-the-counter pain relievers or prescribed medications, if recommended by a healthcare professional, can help manage chronic back pain.

Physical Therapy: Work with a physical therapist to develop tailored exercises and techniques to strengthen the back and alleviate pain.

Lifestyle Modifications for Chronic Back Pain:

Weight Management: Maintain a healthy weight to reduce strain on the back and minimize pressure on the spine.

Healthy Eating: Consume a balanced diet rich in nutrients and anti-inflammatory foods to support overall health and manage pain.

Stress Reduction: Practice stress-relieving techniques like meditation, deep breathing, or mindfulness to reduce tension, which can exacerbate back pain.

Proper Sleep: Ensure quality sleep on a supportive mattress and adopt good sleep hygiene practices for back health.

Integrative Approaches for Chronic Back Pain:

Alternative Therapies: Explore alternative treatments such as acupuncture, chiropractic care, or massage therapy to alleviate back pain.

Mind-Body Techniques: Incorporate relaxation techniques, meditation, or yoga for stress reduction and pain management.

Supportive Devices: Use ergonomic chairs, lumbar cushions, or supportive pillows to maintain proper spinal alignment and reduce discomfort.

Seeking Professional Help:

Healthcare Consultation: Consult a healthcare provider for a personalized treatment plan tailored to manage chronic back pain effectively.

Pain Management Specialists: Consider specialists like pain management doctors or spine specialists for advanced treatment options.

Psychological Support: Seek support from therapists or counselors if chronic pain leads to emotional distress or affects mental well-being.

Conclusion:

Managing chronic back pain involves a multifaceted approach, including lifestyle modifications, physical activity, pain-relieving techniques, and integrative therapies. A comprehensive strategy that combines proper medical guidance, healthy habits, and integrative approaches can significantly improve the management of chronic back pain, enhance overall well-being, and contribute to a better quality of life.

CHAPTER 35

Understanding Herniated Discs:

What is a Herniated Disc?

A herniated disc, also known as a slipped or ruptured disc, occurs when the soft inner material of a spinal disc protrudes through the tough outer layer, pressing on nearby nerves and causing pain.

Causes of Herniated Discs:

Degeneration: Wear and tear on the spinal discs due to aging or repetitive stress can weaken the outer layer, leading to herniation.

Trauma or Injury: Sudden force or injury to the spine, such as lifting heavy objects incorrectly, can cause a disc to herniate.

Genetics: Some individuals may have a genetic predisposition to disc problems, making them more prone to herniated discs.

Symptoms of Herniated Discs:

Back Pain: Pain in the affected area of the spine, which may radiate to the arms or legs, depending on the disc location.

Numbness or Tingling: Numbness, tingling, or weakness in the arms, legs, or feet due to nerve compression.

Muscle Weakness: Weakened muscles or difficulty with fine motor skills in the affected area.

Changes in Reflexes: Altered reflexes in the affected extremity.

Treatment Options for Herniated Discs:

Rest and Activity Modification: Temporary rest followed by gradual return to activities while avoiding strenuous movements that exacerbate pain.

Medications: Over-the-counter pain relievers or prescribed medications to manage pain and reduce inflammation.

Physical Therapy: Specific exercises and stretches to improve strength, flexibility, and alleviate pressure on the affected disc.

Epidural Injections: Steroid injections into the affected area to reduce inflammation and alleviate pain temporarily.

Surgery: In severe cases where conservative treatments fail, surgical procedures like discectomy or spinal fusion may be considered.

Preventive Measures for Herniated Discs:

Proper Lifting Techniques: Lift heavy objects using proper techniques, such as bending the knees and keeping the back straight.

Maintain a Healthy Weight: Excess weight can strain the spine, increasing the risk of disc herniation.

Regular Exercise: Engage in exercises that strengthen core muscles to support the spine and promote overall spine health.

Good Posture: Maintain proper posture while sitting, standing, or lifting to reduce strain on the spine.

Seeking Medical Help:

Healthcare Consultation: Consult a healthcare provider if experiencing persistent back pain, numbness, or weakness.

Diagnostic Tests: Doctors may use imaging tests like MRI or CT scans to confirm a herniated disc diagnosis.

Conclusion:

Herniated discs can cause discomfort and affect daily activities due to nerve compression. Understanding the symptoms, treatment options, preventive measures, and seeking appropriate medical advice can help manage herniated discs effectively, reduce pain, and improve overall spine health for a better quality of life.

CHAPTER 36

Understanding Sciatica Pain:

What is Sciatica?

Sciatica refers to pain that radiates along the path of the sciatic nerve, typically from the lower back through the hips, buttocks, and down one leg.

Causes of Sciatica:

Herniated Disc: Pressure on the sciatic nerve due to a herniated or bulging disc in the spine can cause sciatica.

Bone Spurs: Overgrowth of bone on the vertebrae can compress the nerve, leading to sciatica.

Spinal Stenosis: Narrowing of the spinal canal can result in nerve compression and subsequent sciatic pain.

Piriformis Syndrome: Irritation or compression of the sciatic nerve by the piriformis muscle in the buttocks.

Symptoms of Sciatica:

Radiating Pain: Pain that starts in the lower back or buttocks and travels down the leg, often described as sharp or burning.

Numbness and Tingling: Sensations of numbness, tingling, or weakness in the leg or foot along the nerve pathway.

Muscle Weakness: Weakness in the affected leg that may impact walking or standing.

Worsened Pain with Movement: Pain aggravated by sitting, standing, or sudden movements like sneezing or coughing.

Dealing with Sciatica Pain:

Hot and Cold Therapy: Apply ice packs or heating pads to the affected area to reduce inflammation and alleviate pain.

Medications: Over-the-counter pain relievers or prescribed medications to manage pain and reduce inflammation.

Exercise and Stretching: Gentle exercises and stretches to relieve pressure on the sciatic nerve and improve flexibility.

Physical Therapy: Consult a physical therapist for tailored exercises and techniques to strengthen muscles and reduce pain.

Posture Improvement: Maintain good posture to alleviate pressure on the spine and reduce strain on the sciatic nerve.

Home Care Strategies:

Rest: Take short periods of rest if needed, but avoid prolonged inactivity to prevent muscle stiffness.

Elevate Legs: Elevate legs while lying down to reduce pressure on the nerve and alleviate discomfort.

Supportive Pillows: Use pillows to support the lower back and legs for added comfort while sitting or lying down.

Seeking Medical Help:

Healthcare Consultation: Consult a healthcare provider for persistent or severe sciatica pain.

Diagnostic Tests: Doctors may recommend imaging tests like MRI or CT scans to diagnose the cause of sciatica.

Conclusion:

Dealing with sciatica pain involves a combination of home care strategies, exercises, medications, and seeking medical advice when needed. By understanding the symptoms, employing self-care techniques, maintaining good posture, and seeking appropriate medical help, individuals can effectively manage sciatica pain, reduce discomfort, and improve their quality of life.

CHAPTER 37

Understanding Stress Reduction Techniques:

What is Stress?

Stress is the body's natural response to challenges or demands, often resulting in physical, mental, or emotional strain.

Importance of Stress Reduction:

Impact on Health: Chronic stress can negatively affect overall health, leading to various physical and emotional issues.

Well-being: Reducing stress promotes a sense of calmness, improves mood, and enhances overall well-being.

Improved Coping: Utilizing stress reduction techniques helps in managing challenging situations more effectively.

Stress Reduction Techniques:

Deep Breathing Exercises: Practice deep, slow breathing to calm the body and relax the mind during stressful moments.

Mindfulness and Meditation: Engage in mindfulness practices or meditation to focus attention and reduce mental clutter.

Physical Activity: Regular exercise like walking, yoga, or dancing helps release endorphins, reducing stress and improving mood.

Healthy Lifestyle: Eat a balanced diet, get enough sleep, and limit caffeine or alcohol intake to support stress management.

Time Management: Organize tasks, prioritize activities, and allocate time effectively to reduce feelings of overwhelm.

Relaxation Techniques:

Progressive Muscle Relaxation: Tense and relax different muscle groups to release tension and promote relaxation.

Visualization: Imagine calming scenes or positive outcomes to reduce stress and promote a sense of well-being.

Nature Exposure: Spending time in nature, gardening, or simply enjoying the outdoors can alleviate stress.

Stress Reduction at Work or School:

Take Breaks: Incorporate short breaks during work or study to refresh the mind and reduce stress.

Set Boundaries: Establish clear boundaries between work or school responsibilities and personal time to reduce stress.

Communication: Openly communicate concerns or seek support from supervisors, teachers, or peers when feeling stressed.

Seeking Support:

Social Connections: Connect with friends, family, or support groups to share experiences and receive emotional support.

Professional Help: Consult therapists, counselors, or mental health professionals for guidance in stress management.

Conclusion:

Stress reduction techniques play a vital role in improving mental and physical health by promoting relaxation, improving coping mechanisms, and enhancing overall well-being. By incorporating simple practices like deep breathing, mindfulness, exercise, and maintaining a healthy lifestyle, individuals can effectively manage stress, leading to a more balanced and fulfilling life.

CHAPTER 38

Understanding TENS Units for Back Pain Relief:

What is a TENS Unit?

A TENS (Transcutaneous Electrical Nerve Stimulation) unit is a small, battery-operated device that delivers low-voltage electrical currents to the skin through electrodes placed on the body.

How TENS Units Work:

Pain Gate Theory: TENS units work by stimulating nerves, which may help disrupt pain signals traveling to the brain, essentially "blocking" the sensation of pain.

Endorphin Release: TENS therapy can trigger the release of endorphins, the body's natural pain-relieving chemicals, providing relief.

Using TENS Units for Back Pain:

Application: Electrodes are placed on or near the area of back pain, and the TENS unit is activated to deliver gentle electrical impulses.

Settings and Intensity: Users can adjust the settings, such as intensity and frequency, to suit their comfort level and pain severity.

Duration of Use: TENS sessions typically last around 15-30 minutes, and the device can be used multiple times a day as needed.

Benefits of TENS Units:

Pain Relief: TENS therapy can provide temporary relief from various types of back pain, including muscle soreness, arthritis, or sciatica.

Non-Invasive: TENS units offer a non-invasive and drug-free method for managing pain, reducing the need for medication.

Portable and Convenient: TENS devices are compact and portable, allowing users to use them at home or on the go.

Precautions and Considerations:

Consultation: Seek advice from a healthcare professional before using a TENS unit, especially if pregnant, have a pacemaker, or other medical conditions.

Skin Sensitivity: Ensure clean, dry skin before placing electrodes to avoid skin irritation or discomfort.

Avoid Certain Areas: Avoid using TENS units on certain areas, such as around the eyes, over open wounds, or on the front of the neck.

Effectiveness and Limitations:

Temporary Relief: TENS therapy provides temporary relief and may not be a cure for underlying back conditions.

Varied Results: Effectiveness may vary among individuals, and results may differ based on the cause and severity of back pain.

Conclusion:

TENS units offer a non-invasive, portable, and drug-free option for managing back pain by delivering low-voltage electrical currents. While they can provide temporary relief and offer convenience, it's essential to use TENS units cautiously, following instructions, and seeking guidance from healthcare professionals to ensure safe and effective usage for back pain relief.

CHAPTER 39

Importance of Safety in Exercise:

Exercise Benefits: Regular physical activity brings numerous health benefits, including improved cardiovascular health, strength, flexibility, and mental well-being.

Safety Guidelines for Exercise:

Consultation: Before starting any exercise program, consult a healthcare professional, especially if having health concerns or chronic conditions.

Start Slowly: Begin with low-intensity exercises and gradually increase the intensity and duration to avoid injuries.

Warm-up and Cool-down: Always warm up before exercising to prepare muscles and cool down afterward to prevent muscle strain.

Proper Form: Learn and practice correct exercise techniques to prevent injuries and maximize effectiveness.

Types of Exercises and Safety Tips:

Cardiovascular Exercises:

Safety Tip: Start with moderate-intensity activities like brisk walking or cycling.

Precaution: Avoid overexertion and pace oneself.

Strength Training:

Safety Tip: Use proper equipment and techniques.

Precaution: Gradually increase weight and repetitions to avoid muscle strain.

Flexibility and Stretching:

Safety Tip: Perform gentle stretches after a warm-up or at the end of a workout.

Precaution: Avoid bouncing while stretching to prevent injury.

Safety Equipment and Hydration:

Proper Attire: Wear appropriate clothing and footwear suitable for the exercise activity.

Hydration: Drink water before, during, and after exercising to stay hydrated.

Safety Gear: Use protective equipment like helmets for activities such as cycling or skating.

Listening to Your Body:

Pain: Stop exercising if experiencing severe pain or discomfort and consult a healthcare professional.

Rest: Allow the body to rest between workouts to prevent overtraining and muscle fatigue.

Special Considerations:

Pregnancy: Consult a healthcare provider for safe exercise guidelines during pregnancy.

Age: Tailor exercise routines based on age and fitness level, especially for children and older adults.

Environmental Precautions:

Weather Conditions: Avoid extreme weather conditions like excessive heat or cold during outdoor workouts.

Sun Protection: Use sunscreen and appropriate clothing for protection during outdoor activities.

Conclusion:

Exercising is crucial for overall health, but it's essential to prioritize safety to prevent injuries and achieve maximum benefits. By following safety guidelines, starting gradually, using proper equipment, and listening to the body's signals, individuals can enjoy the positive impacts of exercise while minimizing the risk of injuries or health complications.

CHAPTER 40

Mindful Breathing for Pain Relief:

What is Mindful Breathing?

Mindful breathing involves focusing attention on the breath, using it as an anchor to the present moment, and fostering a sense of calmness and relaxation.

How Mindful Breathing Relieves Pain:

Relaxation Response: Mindful breathing triggers the body's relaxation response, reducing stress and easing pain sensations.

Distraction Technique: Focusing on the breath can distract from the perception of pain, promoting a sense of well-being.

Mindful Breathing Techniques:

Deep Belly Breaths:

Technique: Inhale deeply through the nose, allowing the belly to rise. Exhale slowly through the mouth, letting the belly fall.

Benefits: Deep breathing promotes relaxation, reduces stress, and eases muscle tension, aiding in pain relief.

Counted Breathing:

Technique: Inhale slowly for a count of four, hold the breath for a count of four, exhale slowly for a count of four, and pause for a count of four before inhaling again.

Benefits: Counted breathing helps regulate breathing patterns, calming the nervous system and reducing pain sensations.

Focused Attention:

Technique: Direct attention to the sensation of breathing—feeling the air entering and leaving the body without altering the breath.

Benefits: By focusing on the breath, it promotes mindfulness, reducing the perception of pain and enhancing relaxation.

Practicing Mindful Breathing:

Comfortable Position: Sit or lie down in a comfortable position, ensuring relaxation and minimal distraction.

Quiet Environment: Find a quiet place to practice mindful breathing to enhance focus and relaxation.

Regular Practice: Incorporate mindful breathing into daily routines, especially during moments of pain or discomfort.

Benefits Beyond Pain Relief:

Stress Reduction: Mindful breathing not only alleviates pain but also reduces stress, anxiety, and promotes overall mental well-being.

Improved Focus: Regular practice enhances concentration and focus, fostering a clear and calm mind.

Incorporating Mindful Breathing into Daily Life:

Morning Routine: Start the day with a few minutes of mindful breathing to set a positive tone for the day.

During Activities: Practice mindful breathing during daily tasks or when feeling stressed to regain composure.

Conclusion:

Mindful breathing techniques offer a simple yet powerful approach to pain relief by promoting relaxation, reducing stress, and fostering a calm mind. By incorporating these techniques into daily life, individuals can experience not only relief from pain but also enhanced well-being and a greater sense of control over their health.

CHAPTER 41

Understanding Neuropathic Pain:

What is Neuropathic Pain?

Neuropathic pain is caused by damage or malfunction of nerves, resulting in sensations like shooting, burning, or tingling, often chronic and challenging to treat.

Neuropathic Pain Management:

Medications:

Antidepressants: Certain antidepressants like amitriptyline or duloxetine may help alleviate nerve pain.

Anticonvulsants: Medications used to treat seizures, such as gabapentin or pregabalin, can reduce neuropathic pain.

Topical Treatments:

Lidocaine Patches: Topical patches or creams containing lidocaine can provide localized pain relief.

Capsaicin Cream: Derived from chili peppers, capsaicin creams can help reduce nerve pain when applied topically.

Physical Therapy:

Exercises: Physical therapy includes gentle exercises and stretches to improve mobility and reduce pain.

TENS Therapy: Transcutaneous electrical nerve stimulation (TENS) may help alleviate neuropathic pain.

Nerve Blocks or Injections:

Local Anesthetic Injections: Injecting numbing medications directly into the affected nerve may provide temporary relief.

Nerve Blocks: Blocking specific nerves with injections can help alleviate pain in some cases.

Acupuncture:

Technique: Acupuncture involves inserting thin needles into specific points on the body to alleviate pain.

Benefits: Acupuncture may offer relief for some individuals experiencing neuropathic pain.

Cognitive Behavioral Therapy (CBT):

Therapy Sessions: CBT focuses on changing thought patterns and behaviors related to pain perception.

Benefits: CBT can help manage neuropathic pain by addressing emotional responses to pain.

Lifestyle Modifications:

Regular Exercise:

Low-Impact Activities: Engage in low-impact exercises like swimming or walking to improve circulation and reduce pain.

Healthy Diet:

Nutrient-Rich Foods: A balanced diet with antioxidants and anti-inflammatory foods may help manage pain.

Stress Management:

Relaxation Techniques: Techniques like mindfulness, deep breathing, or yoga can help manage stress, which can exacerbate pain.

Precautions and Considerations:

Consult a Healthcare Provider:

Individualized Treatment: Seek guidance from healthcare professionals for personalized treatment plans.

Medication Side Effects: Discuss potential side effects or interactions of medications with the healthcare provider.

Avoid Self-Medication:

Over-the-Counter Remedies: Avoid self-medicating with over-the-counter medications without consulting a healthcare provider.

Conclusion:

Neuropathic pain management involves a multifaceted approach combining medications, therapies, lifestyle modifications, and professional guidance. While treatments may vary in effectiveness for different individuals, a comprehensive strategy tailored to each person's needs can help improve pain control and quality of life for those experiencing neuropathic pain.

CHAPTER 42

Understanding Dietary Supplements:

What Are Dietary Supplements?

Dietary supplements are products designed to supplement one's diet and can include vitamins, minerals, herbs, botanicals, enzymes, amino acids, or other substances.

Types of Dietary Supplements:

Vitamins and Minerals:

Vitamin Supplements: Common vitamins include Vitamin C, D, E, and B-complex vitamins.

Mineral Supplements: Minerals like calcium, magnesium, iron, and zinc are often available as supplements.

Herbal Supplements:

Popular Herbs: Herbal supplements may include ginseng, turmeric, ginger, or echinacea, among others.

Traditional Uses: Many herbs are used in traditional medicine for various purposes.

Probiotics:

Gut Health: Probiotics contain beneficial bacteria that support digestive health and the immune system.

Omega-3 Fatty Acids:

Source: Omega-3 supplements are derived from fish oil and may promote heart health.

Reasons for Supplement Use:

Nutritional Deficiencies:

Inadequate Diet: Supplements can fill gaps in essential nutrients lacking in one's diet.

Specific Health Conditions:

Addressing Needs: Some supplements are taken to address specific health concerns, like bone health or immunity.

Athletic Performance:

Enhancing Performance: Athletes may use supplements to boost performance or support recovery.

Precautions and Considerations:

Consultation with Healthcare Provider:

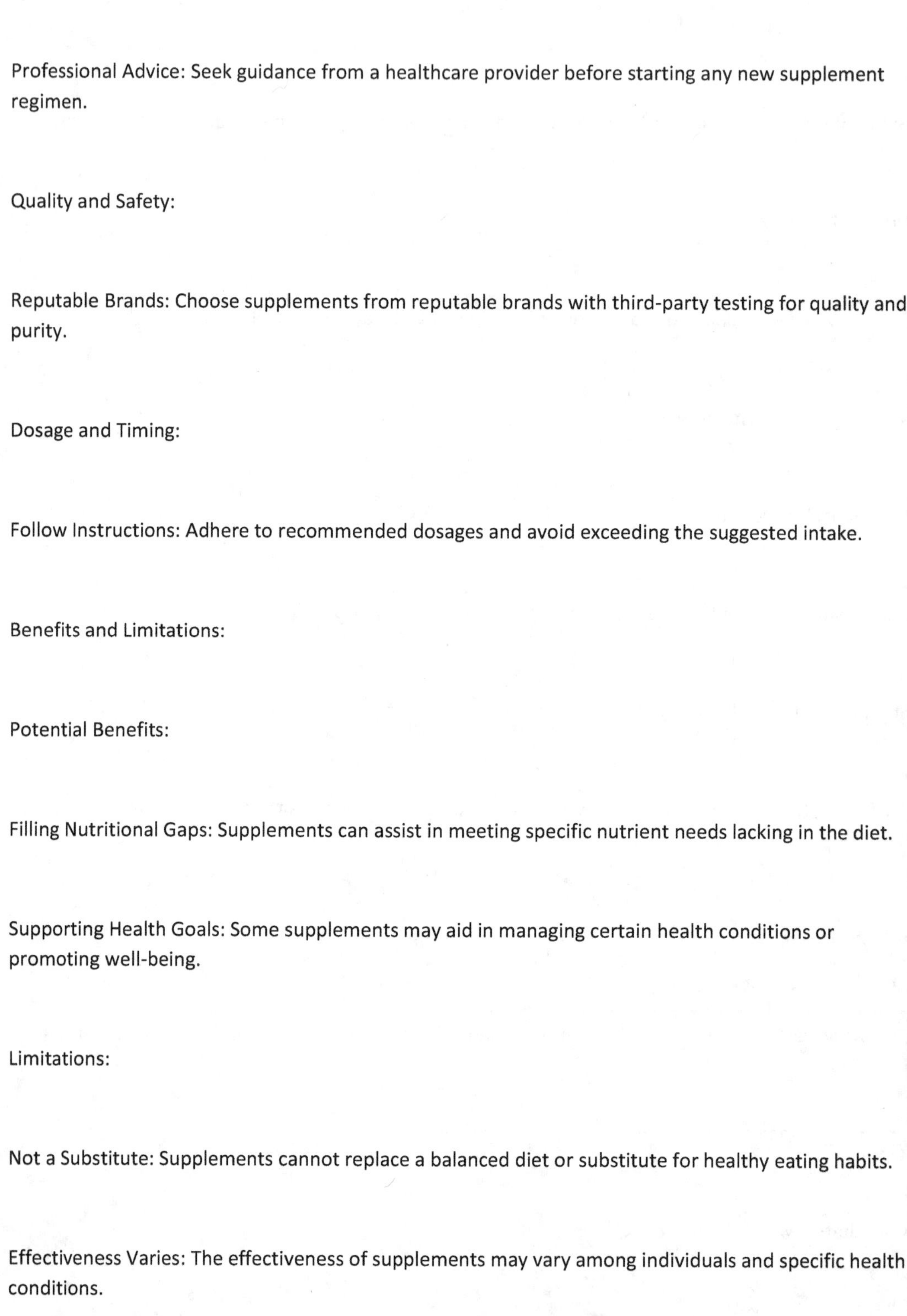

Professional Advice: Seek guidance from a healthcare provider before starting any new supplement regimen.

Quality and Safety:

Reputable Brands: Choose supplements from reputable brands with third-party testing for quality and purity.

Dosage and Timing:

Follow Instructions: Adhere to recommended dosages and avoid exceeding the suggested intake.

Benefits and Limitations:

Potential Benefits:

Filling Nutritional Gaps: Supplements can assist in meeting specific nutrient needs lacking in the diet.

Supporting Health Goals: Some supplements may aid in managing certain health conditions or promoting well-being.

Limitations:

Not a Substitute: Supplements cannot replace a balanced diet or substitute for healthy eating habits.

Effectiveness Varies: The effectiveness of supplements may vary among individuals and specific health conditions.

Conclusion:

Dietary supplements can serve as a helpful addition to support nutritional needs or address specific health concerns. However, they should complement a healthy diet and lifestyle, and individuals should exercise caution by seeking professional guidance, selecting quality products, and understanding that supplements are not a substitute for a balanced diet or medical treatment.

CHAPTER 43

Understanding the Importance of Regular Health Check-Ups:

What are Health Check-Ups?

Health check-ups involve routine examinations, screenings, and consultations with healthcare professionals to monitor and assess overall health status.

Reasons for Regular Health Check-Ups:

Preventive Care:

Early Detection: Check-ups help detect potential health issues before they become severe.

Screenings: Screening tests for various conditions can aid in early diagnosis and timely treatment.

Managing Health Risks:

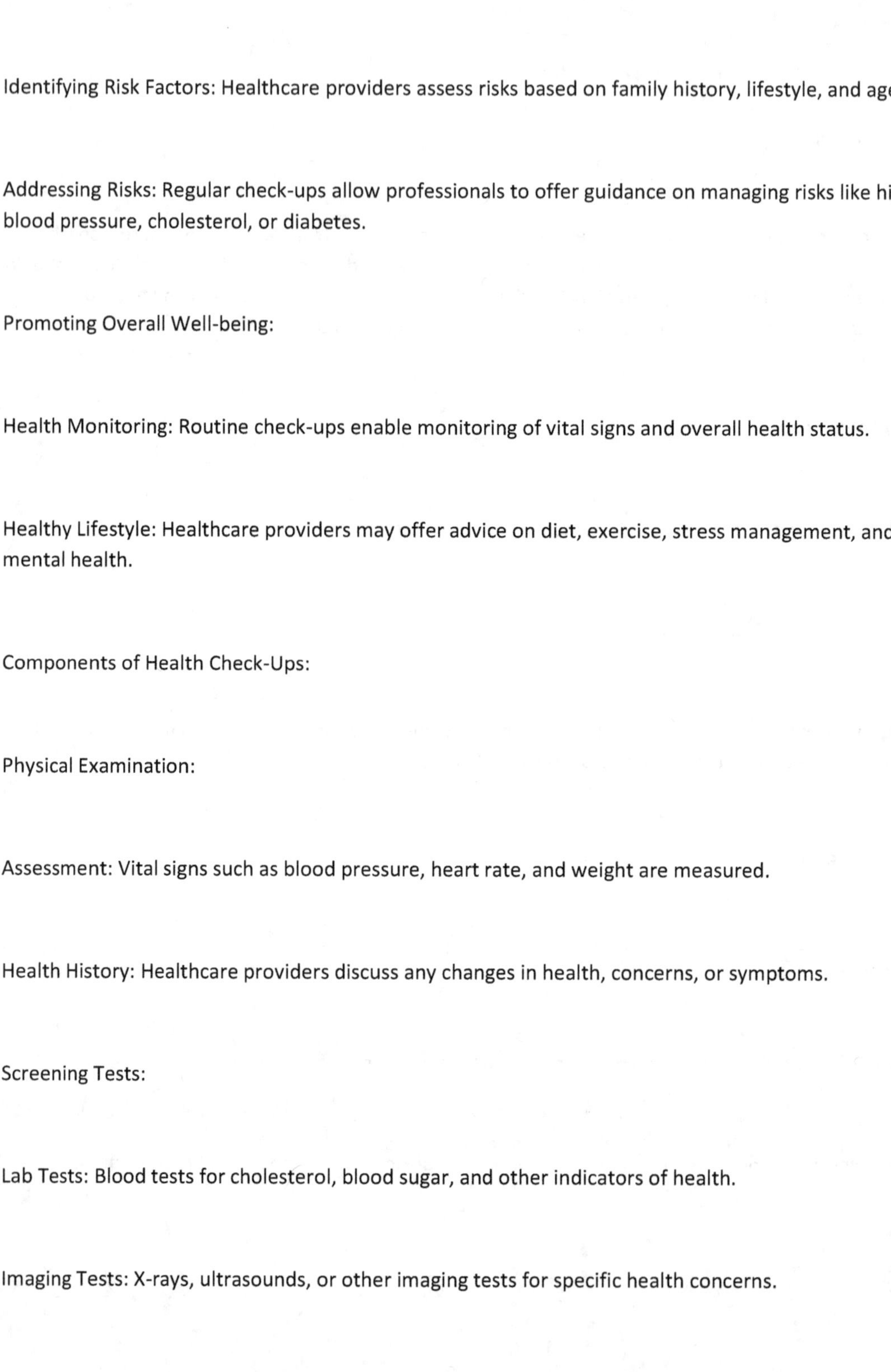

Identifying Risk Factors: Healthcare providers assess risks based on family history, lifestyle, and age.

Addressing Risks: Regular check-ups allow professionals to offer guidance on managing risks like high blood pressure, cholesterol, or diabetes.

Promoting Overall Well-being:

Health Monitoring: Routine check-ups enable monitoring of vital signs and overall health status.

Healthy Lifestyle: Healthcare providers may offer advice on diet, exercise, stress management, and mental health.

Components of Health Check-Ups:

Physical Examination:

Assessment: Vital signs such as blood pressure, heart rate, and weight are measured.

Health History: Healthcare providers discuss any changes in health, concerns, or symptoms.

Screening Tests:

Lab Tests: Blood tests for cholesterol, blood sugar, and other indicators of health.

Imaging Tests: X-rays, ultrasounds, or other imaging tests for specific health concerns.

Health Counseling:

Risk Assessment: Healthcare professionals evaluate lifestyle habits and offer advice for healthier choices.

Preventive Measures: Guidance on vaccinations, cancer screenings, and other preventive measures.

Benefits of Regular Health Check-Ups:

Early Detection and Treatment:

Disease Prevention: Early identification of health issues allows for timely intervention and management.

Improved Outcomes: Addressing health problems in their early stages can lead to better treatment outcomes.

Health Maintenance:

Managing Chronic Conditions: Regular monitoring assists in managing chronic illnesses effectively.

Promoting Healthy Living: Encouragement and guidance for adopting healthy habits.

Frequency of Health Check-Ups:

Age and Health Status:

General Schedule: Frequency may vary based on age, health conditions, and risk factors.

Discuss with Provider: Healthcare professionals can recommend a suitable check-up schedule.

Conclusion:

Regular health check-ups are pivotal for maintaining good health, preventing illnesses, and catching potential health concerns early. They offer an opportunity for individuals to engage with healthcare providers, receive personalized guidance, and take proactive steps towards ensuring overall well-being. By prioritizing regular check-ups, individuals can actively manage their health and improve their quality of life.

CHAPTER 44

Understanding the Balance Between Physical Activity and Rest:

Physical Activity:

Physical activity involves any movement that engages the body's muscles, contributing to overall health and well-being.

Rest:

Rest refers to periods of relaxation or recovery, allowing the body and mind to recuperate from daily activities.

Importance of Balancing Activity and Rest:

Physical Health:

Benefits of Activity: Regular physical activity enhances cardiovascular health, strengthens muscles, and improves flexibility.

Rest and Recovery: Proper rest supports muscle repair, reduces fatigue, and prevents injuries.

Mental Health:

Activity and Mood: Physical activity releases endorphins, promoting feelings of happiness and reducing stress.

Rest and Relaxation: Rest aids in stress reduction, supports mental clarity, and improves overall mood.

Balancing Physical Activity:

Types of Physical Activity:

Aerobic Exercise: Activities like brisk walking, jogging, or cycling.

Strength Training: Using weights or resistance bands to strengthen muscles.

Flexibility Exercises: Stretching and yoga to improve flexibility.

Guidelines for Physical Activity:

Frequency: Aim for at least 150 minutes of moderate-intensity exercise per week.

Variety: Include a mix of aerobic, strength, and flexibility exercises for overall fitness.

Gradual Progress: Start slowly and gradually increase intensity to prevent injuries.

Importance of Rest:

Quality Sleep:

Restorative Sleep: Adequate sleep allows the body to recover, repair, and regenerate tissues.

Sleep Hygiene: Maintain a consistent sleep schedule and create a relaxing bedtime routine.

Recovery from Activity:

Muscle Repair: Rest enables muscles to repair and grow after physical exertion.

Avoiding Overtraining: Adequate rest prevents burnout and overtraining, reducing the risk of injuries.

Strategies for Balancing Activity and Rest:

Listen to Your Body:

Recognize Signs: Pay attention to fatigue, soreness, or signs of exhaustion.

Rest as Needed: Allow for rest days or lighter workouts when feeling fatigued.

Balanced Schedule:

Plan Rest Days: Schedule days for rest or lower-intensity activities within your exercise routine.

Alternate Activities: Alternate between different types of exercises to prevent overuse of specific muscles.

Benefits of Balancing Activity and Rest:

Improved Performance:

Enhanced Fitness: Balanced activity and rest improve physical performance and endurance.

Recovery and Adaptation: Rest helps the body adapt to physical stress and become stronger.

Overall Well-being:

Energy Levels: Balancing activity and rest maintains energy levels throughout the day.

Mental Clarity: Proper rest supports mental focus and concentration.

Conclusion:

Balancing physical activity with adequate rest is crucial for maintaining overall health and well-being. By striking the right balance between exercise and rest, individuals can optimize physical performance, prevent injuries, and ensure mental and physical rejuvenation. Recognizing the importance of both activity and rest in daily routines contributes to a healthier and more balanced lifestyle.

CHAPTER 45

Posture Improvement Through Yoga:

Understanding Posture:

Posture refers to the alignment of the body while sitting, standing, or moving. Good posture involves maintaining the body's natural alignment to prevent strain on muscles and joints.

Importance of Good Posture:

Physical Health:

Spinal Alignment: Good posture supports the spine's natural curvature, reducing back pain.

Muscle Health: Proper alignment eases muscle tension and minimizes strain on ligaments.

Mental Well-being:

Confidence and Mood: Good posture can boost confidence and positively impact mood and self-esteem.

Yoga for Posture Improvement:

Awareness and Alignment:

Mindfulness: Yoga cultivates body awareness, teaching proper alignment and posture.

Core Engagement: Many yoga poses emphasize core strength, which supports better posture.

Stretching and Flexibility:

Lengthening Muscles: Yoga stretches muscles, improving flexibility and releasing tension that impacts posture.

Spine Mobility: Yoga poses encourage gentle spinal movements, enhancing flexibility and mobility.

Yoga Poses for Better Posture:

Mountain Pose (Tadasana):

Benefits: Promotes awareness of standing alignment and engages core muscles for stability.

Downward-Facing Dog (Adho Mukha Svanasana):

Benefits: Stretches the entire body, including the spine, shoulders, and hamstrings.

Cobra Pose (Bhujangasana):

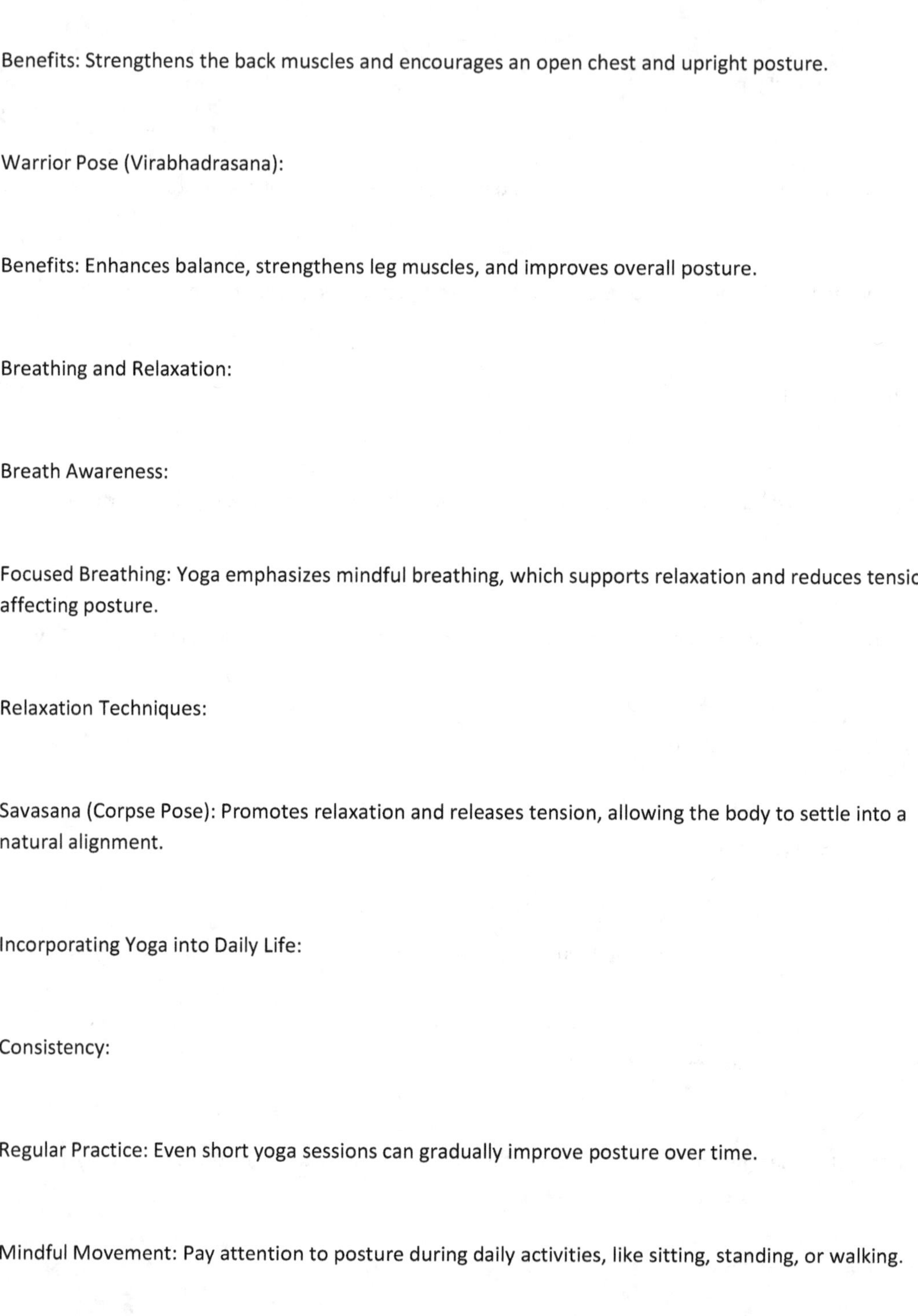

Benefits: Strengthens the back muscles and encourages an open chest and upright posture.

Warrior Pose (Virabhadrasana):

Benefits: Enhances balance, strengthens leg muscles, and improves overall posture.

Breathing and Relaxation:

Breath Awareness:

Focused Breathing: Yoga emphasizes mindful breathing, which supports relaxation and reduces tension affecting posture.

Relaxation Techniques:

Savasana (Corpse Pose): Promotes relaxation and releases tension, allowing the body to settle into a natural alignment.

Incorporating Yoga into Daily Life:

Consistency:

Regular Practice: Even short yoga sessions can gradually improve posture over time.

Mindful Movement: Pay attention to posture during daily activities, like sitting, standing, or walking.

Variety and Adaptability:

Explore Different Poses: Choose poses that target specific areas of concern for posture improvement.

Modify as Needed: Adapt poses to individual comfort levels and physical abilities.

Benefits of Yoga for Posture Improvement:

Strengthening Core Muscles:

Core Stability: Yoga strengthens core muscles, providing a strong foundation for better posture.

Increased Flexibility:

Muscle Lengthening: Improved flexibility reduces stiffness and allows for better alignment.

Mind-Body Connection:

Awareness: Yoga cultivates body awareness, fostering mindful postural adjustments.

Conclusion:

Yoga serves as an effective tool for improving posture by enhancing body awareness, promoting flexibility, and strengthening core muscles. Consistent practice of yoga poses, coupled with mindful breathing and relaxation techniques, can gradually contribute to better posture, reducing discomfort and promoting overall physical well-being. Integrating yoga into daily life can be a valuable step towards maintaining good posture and enjoying its associated benefits.

CHAPTER 46

Understanding Spinal Decompression Therapies:

Spinal Decompression:

Spinal decompression therapies aim to alleviate pain and discomfort in the spine by relieving pressure on the spinal discs, nerves, and surrounding structures.

Importance of Spinal Health:

Spinal Alignment:

Structural Support: A healthy spine provides structural support for the body, aiding movement and stability.

Nerve Function: Proper spinal alignment prevents nerve compression, reducing pain and dysfunction.

Pain Management:

Alleviating Discomfort: Spinal decompression therapies target pain caused by conditions like herniated discs or spinal stenosis.

Types of Spinal Decompression Therapies:

Mechanical Traction Devices:

Equipment-Based: Devices apply traction to stretch the spine gently, reducing pressure on discs and nerves.

Inversion Therapy:

Gravity-Assisted: Inversion tables or chairs use gravity to decompress the spine by hanging upside down.

Manual Decompression Techniques:

Chiropractic Adjustments: Manual manipulation by chiropractors to realign the spine and relieve pressure.

How Spinal Decompression Works:

Reducing Pressure:

Disc Decompression: Traction or inversion allows space between vertebrae, reducing pressure on discs.

Nerve Relief: Alleviating pressure on nerves can reduce pain and tingling sensations.

Promoting Healing:

Improved Blood Flow: Decompression may enhance blood flow to injured areas, aiding healing.

Reduced Inflammation: Relief from pressure may reduce inflammation around spinal discs.

Conditions Treated by Spinal Decompression:

Herniated Discs:

Disc Bulging: Decompression therapies aim to retract herniated discs, reducing pressure on surrounding nerves.

Sciatica:

Nerve Compression: Decompression can alleviate sciatic nerve pain caused by compression.

Degenerative Disc Disease:

Disc Health: May assist in slowing the degenerative process and reducing associated discomfort.

Considerations and Precautions:

Consultation:

Professional Guidance: Seek advice from healthcare providers or specialists before starting decompression therapies.

Suitability: Not all individuals or spinal conditions are suitable for spinal decompression.

Safety Measures:

Proper Use: Follow instructions carefully when using traction devices or inversion tables to prevent injuries.

Monitoring: Regular check-ins with healthcare providers to monitor progress and safety.

Benefits of Spinal Decompression Therapies:

Pain Relief:

Reduced Discomfort: Alleviates back and neck pain associated with spinal conditions.

Improved Mobility: Decreased pain may enhance movement and physical function.

Non-Invasive Approach:

Avoiding Surgery: Offers a non-surgical option for managing certain spinal issues.

Minimized Risks: Generally considered safe with fewer potential risks compared to surgical interventions.

Conclusion:

Spinal decompression therapies aim to alleviate pain and discomfort in the spine by reducing pressure on discs and nerves. While these therapies offer potential relief for various spinal conditions, it's crucial to consult healthcare providers for guidance and determine the suitability of these treatments. Spinal decompression serves as a non-invasive approach to managing pain and promoting spinal health, providing potential relief and improving overall quality of life for individuals experiencing spinal discomfort.

CHAPTER 47

Understanding Chronic Pain Support Groups:

Chronic Pain:

Chronic pain refers to persistent discomfort lasting for an extended period, often affecting one's physical and emotional well-being.

Importance of Support Groups:

Emotional Support:

Sharing Experiences: Groups provide a safe space to discuss challenges and experiences with individuals facing similar issues.

Reducing Isolation: Connects individuals with a supportive community, reducing feelings of loneliness.

Information and Education:

Learning Resources: Groups offer access to information about managing chronic pain through various treatments and coping strategies.

Functions of Support Groups:

Peer Support:

Shared Understanding: Members empathize and understand each other's struggles, offering advice and emotional support.

Validation: Validation from peers can help individuals feel understood and acknowledged.

Coping Strategies:

Skill Sharing: Groups may share coping techniques, relaxation methods, or lifestyle adjustments that help manage pain.

Encouragement: Motivation and encouragement from peers can uplift spirits and promote positivity.

Types of Chronic Pain Support Groups:

In-Person Groups:

Local Meetings: Gatherings held in community centers, hospitals, or designated spaces for face-to-face interaction.

Online Communities:

Virtual Support: Online forums, social media groups, or dedicated websites offering support and information.

Benefits of Support Groups:

Validation and Understanding:

Shared Experiences: Individuals feel understood as they connect with others facing similar challenges.

Reduced Stigma: Diminishes feelings of isolation or judgment often associated with chronic pain.

Emotional Well-being:

Reduced Anxiety: Support groups offer a sense of belonging and reduce anxiety related to chronic pain.

Improved Coping Skills: Learn from others' experiences and gain effective coping strategies.

Participation and Involvement:

Active Involvement:

Contributing Experiences: Sharing personal experiences and insights benefits both individuals and the group.

Seeking Guidance: Asking questions and seeking advice from others fosters a sense of community.

Respectful Environment:

Confidentiality: Groups maintain confidentiality, creating a safe environment for open discussions.

Respectful Interaction: Encourages respect for diverse opinions and experiences within the group.

Finding Support Groups:

Healthcare Providers:

Referrals: Healthcare professionals can recommend local support groups or online communities.

Online Resources:

Directories: Websites or forums dedicated to chronic pain often list available support groups.

Conclusion:

Chronic pain support groups and communities offer valuable emotional support, information, and a sense of community for individuals living with persistent pain. Engaging with these groups provides an opportunity to share experiences, gain coping strategies, and alleviate the emotional burden often associated with chronic pain. Whether through in-person meetings or online platforms, participation in these support networks can significantly impact individuals' emotional well-being, offering a sense of understanding, acceptance, and encouragement in managing chronic pain.

CHAPTER 48

Understanding Visualization and Imagery for Pain Relief:

Visualization and Imagery:

Visualization involves creating mental images or scenarios, while imagery uses the mind to evoke sensory experiences without physical stimuli.

Role in Pain Management:

Mind-Body Connection:

Distraction Technique: Engaging in positive mental imagery can divert attention away from pain sensations.

Brain Response: Imagery may alter brain perception of pain, reducing its intensity.

Emotional Regulation:

Stress Reduction: Visualizing calm scenes or positive experiences can alleviate stress, potentially lessening pain perception.

Emotional Comfort: Imagery promotes relaxation, easing emotional distress linked to pain.

Using Visualization and Imagery:

Guided Imagery:

Scripted Sessions: Listening to a guide narrating calming scenarios to evoke relaxation and pain relief.

Creating Mental Images: Visualizing peaceful scenes or scenarios independently to reduce pain sensations.

Positive Focus:

Pleasant Imagery: Visualizing favorite places, serene landscapes, or happy memories to distract from pain.

Symbolic Imagery: Imagining pain as a color fading away or as a calming river washing discomfort away.

Techniques for Visualization:

Breathing and Relaxation:

Deep Breathing: Pairing visualization with slow, deep breaths to induce relaxation.

Progressive Muscle Relaxation: Combining imagery with muscle relaxation to ease tension and pain.

Sensory Imagery:

Incorporating Senses: Engaging senses (sight, smell, sound) in mental imagery to enhance relaxation.

Vivid Descriptions: Detailed imagery involving colors, textures, and sensations for a more immersive experience.

Steps to Practice Visualization:

Relaxation Preparation:

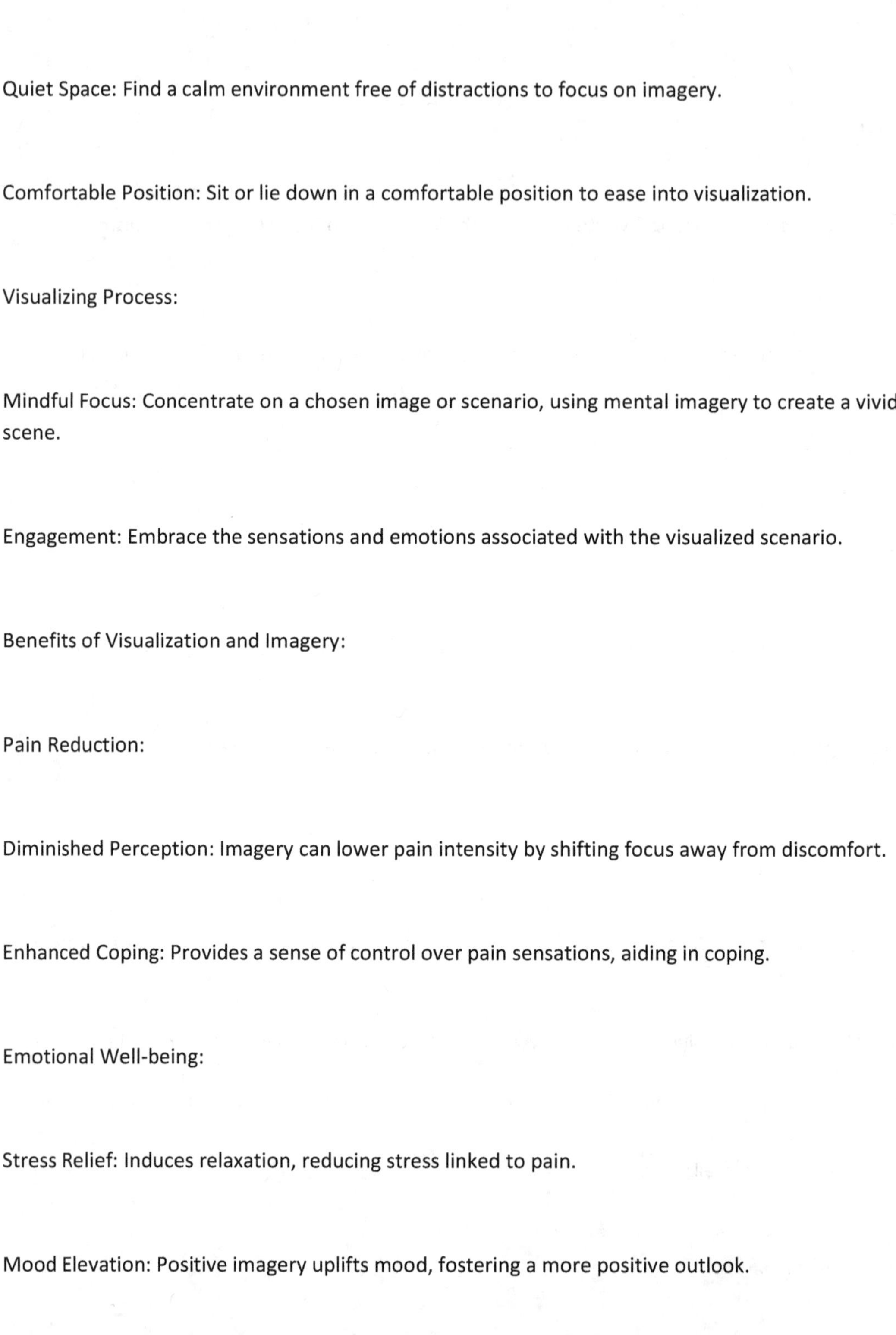

Quiet Space: Find a calm environment free of distractions to focus on imagery.

Comfortable Position: Sit or lie down in a comfortable position to ease into visualization.

Visualizing Process:

Mindful Focus: Concentrate on a chosen image or scenario, using mental imagery to create a vivid scene.

Engagement: Embrace the sensations and emotions associated with the visualized scenario.

Benefits of Visualization and Imagery:

Pain Reduction:

Diminished Perception: Imagery can lower pain intensity by shifting focus away from discomfort.

Enhanced Coping: Provides a sense of control over pain sensations, aiding in coping.

Emotional Well-being:

Stress Relief: Induces relaxation, reducing stress linked to pain.

Mood Elevation: Positive imagery uplifts mood, fostering a more positive outlook.

Conclusion:

Visualization and imagery offer effective tools for managing pain by diverting attention, inducing relaxation, and altering pain perception. Through practice and engagement in guided sessions or personal visualization, individuals can tap into their mind's ability to create calming scenarios, easing both physical discomfort and emotional distress associated with pain. Incorporating visualization and imagery techniques into daily routines can be an empowering aspect of pain management, promoting relaxation and providing relief for individuals experiencing chronic or acute pain.

CHAPTER 49

Understanding Second Opinions and Specialist Referrals:

Second Opinions:

Seeking a second opinion involves consulting another healthcare professional to obtain an additional perspective or assessment regarding a medical condition or treatment plan.

Specialist Referrals:

Specialist referrals occur when a primary care physician recommends or directs a patient to visit a healthcare specialist with expertise in a specific area of medicine.

Importance of Seeking Second Opinions:

Gaining Clarity:

Alternative Insights: Obtaining diverse medical opinions aids in understanding different treatment options.

Validation of Diagnosis: Helps confirm or reevaluate a diagnosis for peace of mind.

Exploring Treatment Options:

Comprehensive Evaluation: Specialists may propose alternative treatments or procedures that align better with individual needs.

Informed Decision-making: Allows patients to make well-informed decisions about their healthcare options.

Reasons for Specialist Referrals:

Expertise and Specialization:

Specific Conditions: Specialists possess in-depth knowledge and experience in treating particular medical conditions.

Complex Cases: For complex or rare conditions requiring specialized care beyond a primary physician's scope.

Diagnostic Clarity:

Precise Diagnosis: Specialists may conduct detailed evaluations or tests to achieve a precise diagnosis.

Process of Seeking Second Opinions and Referrals:

Initiating the Process:

Discussion with Primary Care Provider: Discuss concerns with the primary physician to explore the need for a second opinion or referral.

Referral Requests: Primary care providers can facilitate specialist referrals based on patient needs.

Choosing Specialists:

Research and Recommendations: Research specialists in the required field or ask for recommendations from healthcare professionals.

Insurance Coverage: Consider insurance coverage for specialist visits when making decisions.

Benefits of Seeking Additional Opinions:

Enhanced Decision-making:

Informed Choices: Empowers patients to make informed decisions about their healthcare.

Confidence in Treatment Plan: Increased confidence in chosen treatment plans.

Holistic Care Approach:

Comprehensive Care: Ensures a comprehensive evaluation and potential access to a broader range of treatment options.

Patient-Centered Care: Emphasizes patient preferences and individualized care.

Challenges and Considerations:

Time and Coordination:

Time Investment: Seeking multiple opinions may require additional time and coordination between healthcare providers.

Logistics: Managing appointments, tests, and communications between multiple providers.

Insurance Coverage:

Coverage Limitations: Consider insurance coverage for specialist consultations and any potential out-of-pocket costs.

Conclusion:

Seeking second opinions and specialist referrals are crucial steps in ensuring thorough evaluation, understanding treatment options, and making informed healthcare decisions. These processes enable patients to explore different perspectives, access specialized expertise, and receive comprehensive care tailored to their individual needs. Collaborating with healthcare providers and considering various opinions contributes to a more holistic approach to healthcare, empowering patients to actively participate in their treatment journey and potentially improving health outcomes.

CHAPTER 50

Creating Your Personalized Back Pain Management Plan:

Understanding Back Pain:

Back pain is a common ailment affecting many individuals and can have various causes, including muscle strain, injury, or underlying conditions.

Steps to Develop a Personalized Plan:

Consultation with Healthcare Providers:

Assessment: Discuss concerns with a healthcare provider for a thorough evaluation and accurate diagnosis of the back pain.

Medical History: Share detailed information about medical history, pain symptoms, and any previous treatments.

Understanding Pain Triggers and Patterns:

Identifying Triggers: Recognize activities or situations that worsen or alleviate back pain.

Monitoring Pain Patterns: Keep track of pain levels, triggers, and responses to treatments to identify effective strategies.

Components of a Back Pain Management Plan:

Physical Activity and Exercise:

Tailored Exercise Regimen: Develop an exercise routine focusing on stretching, strengthening, and low-impact aerobic activities.

Guidance from a Professional: Seek advice from a physical therapist or trainer to ensure exercises suit individual needs.

Posture Improvement:

Ergonomic Adjustments: Make ergonomic changes at workstations or home to maintain proper posture and reduce strain on the back.

Awareness of Body Mechanics: Practice good posture and body mechanics during daily activities.

Pain Relief Techniques:

Heat or Ice Therapy: Use heat or ice packs to alleviate pain based on individual preferences or as advised by healthcare providers.

Mind-Body Techniques: Incorporate relaxation methods, such as deep breathing or guided imagery, to manage stress and pain.

Medication Management:

Consultation with a Doctor: Discuss medications suitable for managing back pain, considering over-the-counter or prescribed options.

Adherence to Dosage: Follow prescribed medication instructions carefully to avoid adverse effects.

Healthy Lifestyle Choices:

Nutrition and Weight Management: Maintain a balanced diet and healthy weight to reduce strain on the back.

Adequate Sleep: Prioritize quality sleep to support healing and overall well-being.

Personalizing the Plan:

Individualized Approach:

Consider Specific Needs: Tailor the plan according to individual abilities, preferences, and lifestyle.

Trial and Adaptation: Experiment with different strategies to identify what works best for managing pain.

Communication and Collaboration:

Open Dialogue: Regularly communicate with healthcare providers to discuss progress, modify treatment plans, and address concerns.

Involving Support System: Engage family or friends for support and encouragement in adhering to the management plan.

Long-Term Management and Review:

Consistent Monitoring:

Track Progress: Periodically reassess the effectiveness of the management plan and make necessary adjustments.

Recognize Improvements: Acknowledge improvements in pain levels or functionality achieved through the plan.

Preventive Measures:

Preventing Recurrences: Continue following the plan even after pain subsides to prevent future occurrences.

Precautionary Measures: Be cautious during physical activities to avoid re-injury or exacerbation of back pain.

Conclusion:

A personalized back pain management plan involves a tailored approach that incorporates various strategies to address individual needs and preferences. It's essential to collaborate with healthcare providers, incorporate a range of techniques, maintain healthy lifestyle habits, and adapt the plan as necessary. By understanding personal triggers, consistently following the plan, and making necessary adjustments, individuals can effectively manage their back pain and improve their overall quality of life.

* Please note that managing back pain is highly individualized, and what works for one person might not work for another. Always consult with healthcare professionals to determine the most suitable approaches for your specific condition.